Social Work and Intimate Partner Violence

Intimate partner violence is now recognised as a serious human rights abuse and increasingly as an important public health problem with severe consequences for women's physical, mental and sexual health. Therefore, a comprehensive understanding of intimate partner violence is an essential aspect of good-quality social work practice. This is an accessible introduction to the complexities of social work practice with abused women, as well as men.

Designed for those new to practice in this area, it outlines and explores some of the key issues from an international perspective, such as the role and responsibilities of a social worker, prevalence rates and research around causes and consequences. It includes chapters on working with women with additional vulnerabilities, working with perpetrators, impacts on physical and mental health, child protection issues, assessment and intervention strategies, and long-term approaches.

Social Work and Intimate Partner Violence is an up-to-date book bringing together all the most important information in the area for social workers, and is essential reading for all students and newly qualified professionals.

Mary Allen is Lecturer in Social Work at University College Dublin, Ireland.

Social Work and Intimate Partner Violence

Mary Allen

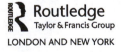

Routledge
Taylor & Francis Group

LONDON AND NEW YORK

First published 2013
by Routledge
2 Park Square, Milton Park, Abingdon, Oxon OX14 4RN

Simultaneously published in the USA and Canada
by Routledge
711 Third Avenue, New York, NY 10017

Routledge is an imprint of the Taylor & Francis Group, an informa business

British Library Cataloguing in Publication Data
A catalogue record for this book is available from the British Library

Library of Congress Cataloging-in-Publication Data
Allen, Mary.
  Social work and intimate partner violence / Mary Allen.
    p. cm.
  1. Family violence.   2. Family violence—Prevention.
  3. Family social work.   4. Victims of family violence—Services for.
  5. Child welfare.   I. Title.
  HV6626.A425 2013
  362.82'9253—dc23   2012036189

ISBN: 978-0-415-51838-3 (hbk)
ISBN: 978-0-415-51840-6 (pbk)
ISBN: 978-0-203-38766-5 (ebk)

Typeset in Times New Roman
by RefineCatch Limited, Bungay, Suffolk

Contents

Illustrations

Figures

Tables

1 Introduction

Domestic violence, also known as intimate partner violence, is an issue which has been seen to be problematic within social work practice. Social workers, as will be seen later in this book, tend to make decisions on child protection without making assessments of whether or not domestic violence is a factor in their abuse. It is now known that there is an important overlap between such abuse and the abuse of children. Social workers in health and mental health settings also encounter such abuse. However, there is serious criticism of how social workers deal with this abuse, how they understand it, and the extent to which they focus on child protection rather than woman protection. This textbook will explore the many controversies surrounding this serious issue. It will examine the emphasis social workers place on child protection, the lack of consistent assessment guidelines, the emerging belief that abuse by women is equal to that perpetrated by men, women at greatest risk of abuse, the risk of femicide (the murder of women, usually in situations of domestic abuse) and the impact of perpetrator programmes. Such issues need to be understood by social workers in practice, and by their managers, as their responses to such abuse will impact on both women's and children's safety. Acquiring a comprehensive understanding of violence against women is an essential aspect of good quality social work practice, whether this practice is carried on within the child protection sector, or within other social work areas.

Adult intimate violence against women

Terminology

Violence against women is an interpersonal experience which has been, over the centuries and across cultures, in turn condoned, tolerated, denied, stigmatised, pathologised, and criminalised. It has also been renamed, from wife battering to domestic violence, spousal abuse to intimate partner violence, each 'name' representing a reframing of this private experience within the public consciousness. Each title used to describe this private experience carries with it a range of implications, emphasising one or more aspects of the experience. For example 'woman battering' implies an emphasis on physical 'battering'. 'Spousal abuse' broadens the concept of abuse, but narrows the context of the relationship of the parties concerned to that between legally married partners.

The terms 'family abuse/violence', 'domestic violence' and 'spousal assault' are used differently in different countries and the meaning is different, particularly in relation to gender. The term 'family violence' implies that all members of the family are engaged in mutual conflict, while the term 'spousal abuse' excludes women who are co-habiting or in dating relationships and women who are abused by their sons or fathers. The term 'battering' obscures the fact that abuse can also be emotional, sexual, psychological or economic (Allen and Perttu, 2010). The World Health Organization (WHO) also notes that when abuse occurs repeatedly in the same relationship, the phenomenon is often referred to as 'battering' (Krug *et al*. 2002). 'Family violence' is a generic term that encompasses elder abuse, child abuse, and intimate partner violence (American Medical Association, AMA, 2005).

The American Medical Association (AMA) defines intimate partner abuse as 'the physical, sexual, and/or psychological abuse to an individual perpetrated by a current or former intimate partner'. The AMA also notes it as 'past or present physical and/or sexual violence between former or current intimate partners, adult household members, or adult children and a parent. Abused persons and perpetrators could be of either sex, and couples could be heterosexual or homosexual' (Sugg *et al.*, 1999).

While the term 'intimate partner abuse' is gender neutral, women are more likely to experience physical injuries and incur psychological consequences of intimate partner abuse. The gendered nature of this crime is indicated by the fact that worldwide research in many arenas has shown that between 90% and 97% of abusive incidents within an intimate relationship are perpetrated by men against women (this will be discussed in greater detail in Chapter 3). For this reason the terms 'domestic violence' or 'spousal abuse' are misnomers as they obscure the gender of the perpetrator and that of the victim.

'Domestic violence' is undoubtedly the most commonly used title in recent years (McWilliams and McKiernan, 1993) yet this can include abuse between members of a domestic unit other than heterosexual or homosexual intimate partners. The title 'adult intimate abuse' overcomes this overly broad definition, yet does not limit the direction of the abuse to heterosexual partners, and does not indicate the 'directionality' (Forgey and Badger, 2006) of such abuse. Hammons (2004: 280) notes that a term such as 'violence against women' indicates that it is structural inequality between men and women that is the key factor in this form of violence. Radford (2003: 34) argues that it is important to avoid overly broad definitions as this can result in the minimisation of domestic violence through its reconstruction as an 'equal opportunities crime'. It may therefore be unrealistic to expect one relatively short and readily usable title to capture fully such a complex issue. For the purposes of this textbook, therefore, the titles 'domestic violence', 'intimate partner violence', 'adult intimate abuse', 'adult intimate violence against women' will be used interchangeably to name the experience of physical, sexual and emotional abuse, as well as the coercive control of women by their intimate male partners in a heterosexual relationship. The limiting of the focus of this study to violence against heterosexual women does not imply that intimate partner violence only occurs between heterosexual partners, or is always male to female in direction. The debates and complexities surrounding these issues will be reviewed in detail in Chapter 2.

Definitions of domestic violence

Just as the title used to name the experiences of intimate partner or domestic abuse has varied over time and across important literature in the field, the definition of what exactly is being referred to has also varied. One of the most important definitions of violence against women is that outlined in the 1995 *Beijing Declaration and Platform of Action* as it is both 'gendered and culturally sensitive':

> The term 'violence against women' means any act of gender-based violence that results in, or is likely to result in, physical, sexual or psychological harm or suffering to women, including threats of such acts, coercion or arbitrary deprivation of liberty, whether occurring in public or private life. Accordingly, violence against women encompasses but is not limited to the following:
>   a. Physical, sexual and psychological violence occurring in the family, including battering, sexual abuse of female children in the household, dowry-related violence, marital rape, female genital mutilation and other traditional practices harmful to women . . .
>
> (UN, 1995: 73–74)

This definition encompasses a range of abuses towards women including female genital mutilation. It is a broader definition than one which focuses only on abuse within an adult intimate relationship. While it includes physical and emotional abuse it does not refer to the range of coercive behaviours which it is now recognised is at the heart of domestic abuse.

In view of the influence of the *Report of the Task Force on Violence Against Women* (1997), from the Office of the Tanaiste (Office of the Deputy Prime Minister) on Irish policy making in this field, it will be helpful to also cite the definition chosen by the Task Force in its examination of the issue:

> The use of physical or emotional force or the threat of physical force, including sexual violence in close adult relationships. It can also involve emotional abuse; the destruction of property; isolation from friends, family and other potential sources of support; threats to others including children; stalking; and control over access to money, personal items, foods, transportation and the telephone.
>
> (*Report of the Task Force on Violence Against Women*, 1997)

This definition highlights that violence against women is not only about physical violence, but also includes sexual and emotional abuse. It also highlights that the control of the partner's actions, such as isolating her from family and friends, preventing her from working outside the home, and keeping close track over money and the use of the telephone is another important aspect of violence against women. Since this definition was published smartphones can now also be used to track women and ensure that their partners know where they are all day. This use of this new technology has added to women's sense of powerlessness and has subjected them to even greater daily surveillance.

International organisations such as the United Nations (UN) and the European Union (EU) have also defined domestic violence. The UN Secretary-General's *In-depth Study on Violence Against Women* (2006) defines gender-based violence against women as 'violence that is directed against a woman because she is a woman, or violence that affects women disproportionately. It includes physical, mental or sexual harm or suffering, threats of such acts, coercion and other deprivations of liberty'. This definition also includes coercion and the deprivation of liberty, as well as physical mental and sexual abuse.

The definition of violence against women by the EU is based on the UN *Declaration on the Elimination of Violence against Women* (1993). The EU emphasises the human rights and gender equality-based approach to violence against women and points out that the obstacles to exercising women's socio-economic and political rights increase women's exposure to violence. The EU notes that violence against women is a manifestation of the historically unequal power relations between men and women and adversely affects not only women but society as a whole, and therefore urgent action is required. Joint actions by public authorities, institutions, and society in general, as well as an integral and multidisciplinary approach, are necessary for the eradication of violence against women (Allen and Perttu, 2010).

The Council of Europe seeks to develop throughout Europe common and democratic principles-based on the European Convention on Human Rights (Council of Europe, 1950). It gave the following declaration in 1993: 'Violence against women constitutes an infringement of the right to life, security, liberty and dignity of the victim and, consequently, a hindrance to the functioning of a democratic society, based on the rule of law'.

Violence against women is now recognised as a serious human rights abuse and increasingly as an important public health problem with serious consequences for women's physical, mental, sexual and reproductive health (Garcia-Moreno *et al.*, 2006). In all member countries of the EU, violence against an intimate partner, or against children, is a crime punishable by imprisonment or other legal sanctions.

Coker *et al.*'s (2003) definition, (which is gender neutral), also emphasises the loss of power and control by one partner because of the actions of the other partner:

A process whereby one member of an intimate relationship experiences vulnerability, loss of power and control and entrapment as a consequence of the other member's exercise of power through the patterned use of physical, sexual, psychological and/or moral force.

(Coker *et al.*, 2003: 260)

This definition also emphasises that domestic violence is not only about physical violence, but is primarily about the use of power and control over women. The Duluth Model is an excellent example of the use of this approach to domestic violence. This model (see Figure 1.1) was drawn up by the female partners of men in their perpetrator programme, and is now used internationally as a template of what domestic violence is primarily about (Pence and Paymar, 1993).

This range of behaviours encompasses the spectrum of control and abuse that women are subjected to in domestically violent relationships. These tactics include isolating the woman from her family and friends, treating her like a servant, making all the decisions about money in the family, using emotional abuse such as telling her what to wear or whether or not to allow her to use make up, threatening to abuse her, or to leave her or commit suicide. Abusing pets is another means of evoking distress for the woman and the children. A study carried out by Allen *et al.* (2007) in a number of women's refuges found that 57% of women and 50% of children reported witnessing one or more forms of abuse, or threats of abuse, of their pets. Threats reported included neglect, physical abuse to kill the pet, while abuse also

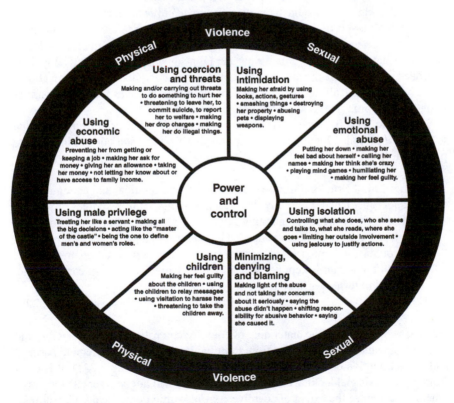

Figure 1.1 The Duluth Model Power and Control Wheel.

Source: Pence and Paymar, 1993. Reproduced with permission.

included neglect of their basic needs and/or a variety of physical assaults, five of which were reported to result in the death of the pet. This overlap of abuse of pets and domestic violence is another indicator of the extent of such abuse in family homes. Making light of the abuse is also a common occurrence, as is blaming the woman for the abuse. Using the children is one of the issues that many social workers do not often recognise – threatening to abuse them if the woman doesn't do what her partner wants, or threatening to take them from their mother. In their work Pence and Paymar (1993) outline that these tactics are part of a pattern of behaviours rather than isolated incidents of abuse or cyclical explosions of pent-up anger, frustration or painful feelings. A batterer's use of physical assaults or sexual abuse is often infrequent, but it reinforces the power of the other tactics on the wheel (emotional abuse, isolation, threats to take the children) that are used at random and eventually undermine his partner's ability to act autonomously (Pence and Paymar, 1993: 2).

The National Crime Council's Irish Prevalence study (Watson and Parsons, 2005) defined severe domestic abuse as 'a pattern of physical, emotional or sexual behaviour between partners in an intimate relationship that causes, or risks causing, significant negative consequences for the person affected'.

They go on to state that it is behaviour (not just a single act) in intimate relationships of the kind that would have significant negative impact (either physical injury, or high levels of distress) on the person affected. These acts rarely occur in isolation: those experiencing severe abuse generally suffer a number of different types of behaviour from the abusive partner (Watson and Parsons, 2005: 23). This approach to such abuse mirrors the work of Pence and Paymar (1993) cited above. It is a range of controlling and abusive behaviour which leaves the abused partner (usually the woman) without control of her own life.

Evan Stark's (2007) recent work *Coercive Control: How Men Entrap Women in Personal Life* also highlights the importance of power and control in intimate partner violence. He defines control as:

> comprised of structural forms of deprivation, exploitation, and command that compel obedience indirectly by monopolizing vital resources, dictating preferred choices, microregulating a partner's behaviour, limiting her options, and depriving her of supports needed to exercise independent judgement. . . . Control may be implemented through specific acts of prohibition or coercion, as when the victim is kept home from work, denied access to a car or phone, or forced to turn over her paycheck.
>
> (Stark, 2007: 229)

He goes on to state that 'the materiality of coercive control refers to the tangible and symbolic advantages men accrue from dominating and exploiting female partners and the substantive deprivations that women suffer' (Stark, 2007: 231). It is clear from his analysis that looking only at physical abuse will not help social workers or others to recognise the extent of coercive control within domestically violent relationships. Utilising assessment tools which can identify such control is essential to fully understanding the nature of such control and its impact on women victims.

Working from these broad and comprehensive definitions, the prevalence of the problem of violence against women will be examined from an international perspective.

Prevalence of intimate partner violence

International prevalence

The WHO estimates that between 10% and 69% of women worldwide experience physical violence at the hands of intimate partners and up to 70% of female murder victims are killed by their male partners (Heise and Garcia-Moreno, 2002: 89–93).

The more recent WHO multi-country study (Garcia-Moreno *et al.*, 2006) established the prevalence figures for 15 sites in 10 countries internationally. Of those women who reported experiencing either physical or sexual violence by an intimate partner, the highest rate, 71%, was found in Butajira, in the south of Ethiopia, and the lowest rate was found in Japan, at 15%. The other countries in the study included Bangladesh (city rate was 53.4% and provincial rate was 61.7%), Brazil (city rate was 28.9% and provincial rate was 36.9%), Namibia city, where the rate was 35.9%, Peru (city rate was 51.2% provincial rate was 69%), Samoa, where the rate was 42.1%, Serbia and Montenegro city, where the rate was 20.7%, Thailand (city rate was 41.1% and provincial rate was 47.4%), the United Republic of Tanzania, in which the rates were 41.3% in the city and 55.9% in the rural province. As can be seen from these figures, the provincial rates were always higher than the city rates. As Garcia-Moreno *et al.* (2006: 1265) note, most acts of physical partner violence were part of a pattern of continuing abuse. They also suggest that these figures are likely to be an underestimate as women are commonly stigmatised and blamed for the abuse they receive.

Studies in a number of African countries also report high rates of intimate partner abuse. A number of studies from the sub-Saharan African region have found that violence against women is widespread (Mann and Takyi, 2009). These studies have found approximately half of all married women in Zambia, 57% in Uganda, 60% in Tanzania, 42% in Kenya, 67% in Sierra Leone, and 81% in Nigeria have experienced some form of violence in their lives from partners or husbands (Coker *et al.*, 2003; Heise *et al.*, 1999; Kishor and Johnson, 2004; Mann and Takyi, 2009; Speizer, 2010). Studies in South Africa have suggested that violence against women is 'endemic' to South African society (Vogelman and Eagle, 1991). The South African Police Service estimated that 80% of women living in rural areas are victims of abuse (cited in Boonzaier and de La Rey, 2003).

The United Nations Population Fund Report (2000) states that one in three women have been beaten, coerced into sex or abused in some way, and mostly by a male intimate partner or family member. One in four women have been abused during pregnancy.

In the USA more than 1 million cases of intimate partner violence are reported to police each year (Goldberg, 1999). The National Coalition Against Domestic

Violence reports that on average 10 women die at the hands of intimate partners each day (Wood, 2001). In Canada, there were 28,000 incidents of spousal violence reported to the police in 2004, of which 84% involved female victims and 16% involved male victims. However, only 28% of spousal abuse victims report incidents to the police (36% of female victims and 17% of male victims (Ogrodnik, 2006).

Prevalence in some European countries

The EU estimates that at some point in their lives, 1 in 5 European women will experience abuse by a male partner, while 25% of all reported crime involves assaults by a man on his wife or partner (EU, 2007). It is the major cause of death and disability for women aged between 16 and 44, accounting for more death and illness than cancer and road traffic accidents (Council of Europe, 2002). Partner violence accounts for a high proportion of homicides of women internationally. Between 40% and 70% of female murder victims were killed by their partners or former partners. The comparably figure for men is 4–8% (Krug *et al.*, 2002).

Since the 1980s a number of European countries have conducted major nation-wide statistical surveys on the extent of interpersonal violence and its impact. The extent of the problem is recognised, and many countries have taken actions to address the issue. Still there is a need for European data so that social and political interventions can be effectively targeted and tailored to meet the current needs. Comparative data can advance theory and suggest improvements to cultural, political and societal responses to violence. However, accurate data comparison is more difficult than it seems. Ignoring or misjudging the scientific and methodological framework of specific data easily leads to wrong conclusions and interpretations. There have been attempts to compare prevalence data but they have faced many problems and data comparison has sometimes been impossible (Allen and Perttu, 2010).

A European research network called Coordination Action on Human Rights Violations (CAHRV) has addressed these problems and has taken the first steps to review European surveys on the prevalence and health impact of violence against women. Results show that the studies are constructed quite differently from one country to the next, and neither prevalence nor health impact data are comparable on a European level.

The report introduces the national violence against women surveys in Finland, France, Germany, Lithuania and Sweden. In those surveys there are differences and similarities of sample size and age range, data collection methods and year of the surveys.

Lifetime prevalence rates for physical violence by current and/or former partners range from almost 21% to 33% for women in the central age group of 20–59 who ever had a partner in Finland, Germany, Lithuania or Sweden. The French survey collected data on prevalence only in the past 12 months. Prevalence of physical violence by a current or former partner over the past 12 months ranges from 3% in Germany and France to 5% in Sweden and 7% in Finland. The Lithuanian survey did not include questions on last-year-prevalence. The age group of women between 20 and 59 reported high levels of lifetime prevalence of sexual violence by current and/or former partners, with 11.5% in the Finnish study, 6.5% in Germany, 7.5% in the Lithuanian and 6.2% in the Swedish study.

It is difficult to define exactly what is psychological violence in intimate partner relationships. Most prevalence studies use several dimensions of dominance, humiliating behaviour, threats and control in order to measure psychological violence. Indicators that were assessed in the Swedish, Finnish, Lithuanian, German, and, to some extent, in the French surveys were extreme jealousy, restricting the woman from seeing friends or relatives, humiliating behaviour, economic control, threats to harm the children and threats of suicide. In the Lithuanian study at least one of these partner behaviours of the current partner was reported by 28.6% of women, and the percentages were 24.3% in the French study, 16.5 % in the Finnish study, 14.3% in Germany and 11.6% in the Swedish study (Schröttle *et al.*, 2006). A study in Iceland established that 22% of women had experienced domestic violence at some point in their lives. Of these women, 26% said they were in danger of their lives, and 41% were physically injured. Only 13% of abused women contacted the police (NIKK).

UK and Irish prevalence rates

In Britain, one in four women will be a victim of domestic violence in their lifetime (Mirrlees-Black, 1999). One incidence of domestic violence is reported to the police every minute (Stanko, 2000), and it is the crime with the highest repeat victimisation rate in Britain (Kewshaw *et al.*, 2000). An average of two women per week are killed by a male partner or former partner, and nearly half of all female murder victims are killed by a partner or ex-partner (Coleman *et al.*, 2006). The 2001 British Crime Survey found that 45% of women and 26% of men aged 16–59 reported having experienced domestic violence (abuse, threats or force), sexual victimisation or stalking at least once in their lifetimes, and those who suffer multiple attacks are more like to be women (Walby and Allen, 2004: vi,11). The findings of the Domestic Violence Matters Evaluation Study strongly confirm the gendered nature of domestic and intimate partner abuse. Of the 1,236 individuals with whom the civilian support workers worked within the context of the British police system, 99% of the service users were female and 99% of the perpetrators were male (Kelly *et al.*, 1999).

According to Women's Aid in England, their National Freephone Domestic Violence helpline received over a quarter of a million calls during its first 12 months. Domestic violence accounts for between 16% and 25% of all recorded violent crime (Home Office, 2004). In any one year there are 13 million separate incidents of physical violence or threats of violence against women from partners or former partners. In the UK 54% of rapes are committed by a woman's current or former partner (Walby and Allen, 2004), and two women per week are killed by a male partner or former partner (Povey, 2004).

Irish prevalence studies

To date there have been only two national prevalence studies on domestic violence carried out in Ireland. The first of these, *Making the Links* (Kelleher and Associates, 1995), was commissioned by the national voluntary campaigning and service organisation, Women's Aid. The study, which randomly selected 1,483 women (aged 18 years or over) nationwide, of whom 679 (46%) responded, found that 18% of women who had ever been in an intimate relationship with a man had experienced abuse of either a physical, sexual or emotional nature. Emotional abuse was experienced by 13%, 10% had experienced actual physical abuse, 9% threats of such abuse, while 4% reported sexual abuse and assault, and 2% had their property damaged. The study also included an area-based survey in North Dublin, in which they distributed confidential questionnaires to women attending six general practitioners' surgeries, of which 240 were completed. In this smaller sample, 36% of those who had ever been in an intimate relationship had experienced violence of a physical or emotional nature.

The second and most recent prevalence study, *Domestic Abuse of Women and Men in Ireland* (Watson and Parsons, 2005), was commissioned by the National Crime Council and carried out by the Economic and Social Research Institute. In response to recent academic and other commentary regarding the abuse of men within intimate relationships (Steinmetz, 1977/8; Straus *et al.*, 1980; Straus and Gelles, 1990; McKeown and Kidd, 2003; Archer, 2000) this 2005 study set out to be gender neutral in its sampling and analysis, surveying both men and women on their experiences of abuse within an intimate relationship. A nationally representative sample of 3,077 men and women were surveyed by telephone about their lifetime victimisation experiences in relation to intimate partner violence. Respondents were asked if they had been subjected to specific acts of physical, sexual or emotional abuse, how frequently the acts had occurred and the physical and/or psychological impact of these acts. The analysis distinguishes between minor and severe abuse, defining the latter as 'a pattern of physical, emotional or sexual behaviour between partners in an intimate relationship that causes, or risks causing, significant consequences for the person affected' (Watson and Parsons, 2005: 23). When looking at the prevalence of either severe or minor incidents of any form of abuse, 29% of the women and 26% of the men had experienced some form of abuse (at some point in their lives). Combining the figures for physical abuse alone, of both a minor and severe nature, 13% of women and men had experienced either minor or severe abuse.

Using the definition of severe abuse alone, the study found a 15% lifetime prevalence of severe intimate partner abuse for women and 6% for men: 1 woman in 11 had experienced severe physical abuse, 1 in 12 severe sexual abuse, and 1 in 13 severe emotional abuse. This figure of 15% is somewhat lower than the 18% found in *Making the Links* (Kelleher and Associates, 1995).

The study also identified a number of factors which increased the risk of experiencing domestic abuse (Watson and Parsons, 2005: 24–25):

- being female (women were over twice as likely to experience physical abuse, and seven times more likely to experience sexual abuse);
- being young (for women the risk of experiencing abuse declined 15% every 10 years);
- having parents who were abusive to each other (for both women and men, this doubled the risk of being abused);
- not being allowed to make decisions about money in the relationship (the risk of severe abuse increased sevenfold for women whose partners controlled the decision making about money);
- having children (the risk increased threefold for women who had ever had children);
- being isolated from family and neighbourhood support (the risk increased by 27% for those living in an urban rather than a rural area, and by 75% for those born outside Ireland).

Women's Aid in Ireland reported that in 2010, 13,575 incidents of domestic violence were reported to their Freephone helpline. These included 8,351 incidents of emotional abuse, 3,031 incidents of physical abuse and 1,605 incidents of financial abuse. There were also 588 incidents of sexual abuse disclosed, including 213 rapes (*National and International Statistics*, 2012). In a one day survey in November 2010, 555 women and 324 children were accommodated and/or received support from a domestic violence service; 140 helpline calls were received from women; 108 women were accommodated in refuges and 98 women in transitional housing (Safe Ireland, 2011). Safe Ireland also found that in one year, over 3,000 women were unable to access a refuge when they needed it, as either the refuges were full or there were no refuges in their area.

Conclusion

This chapter has outlined some of the definitions of domestic violence and intimate partner violence. As can be seen from these definitions, the issue of coercive control and power is becoming more central to these definitions. Understanding domestic violence only as a form of physical violence will lead many professionals to misunderstand this form of abuse. As noted by Watson and Parsons (2005), it is a pattern of behaviour, not one-off incidents, which is motivated by the need to exert power and dominance over one's partner.

Without such an understanding of the pervasive and sometimes hidden forms of control, it will not be possible to make correct assessments or provide abused women with the support they need. The statistics cited from many international sources also make it clear that such abuses of women are not isolated events but in fact are extremely common, and require a thorough understanding of the issues involved in order to respond appropriately and effectively. Many professionals accept some of the myths surrounding this form of abuse, and these myths (listed below) will be discussed in the following chapters of this textbook.

Myths about intimate partner violence

- Only a small percentage of women are victims of violence.
- Nobody has the right to interfere in the domestic affairs of a couple.
- Women deserve to get raped and beaten; they provoke the assault by their behaviour and clothing.
- It's just the odd domestic tiff – not as bad as they make out.
- Physical violence is unlikely to get worse over time.
- Only poor women are abused.
- If there were no visible injuries then the assault cannot have been that bad.
- Nobody ever gets killed as a result of domestic violence.
- Battered women can always leave home if they want to.
- Women who are abused come from an abusive family background.
- Battering only occurs in working class and ethnic minority families.
- If a woman leaves the abusive relationship the abuse will stop.
- Women who experience domestic violence are weak.
- Alcohol misuse causes wife battering.
- Couple counselling will help resolve the abuse.
- Women and children frequently lie about sexual violence.
- Battered women batter their children.
- Violent men are mentally ill or have low self-esteem.
- Men who are violent come from an abusive family background.
- Abusive men cannot control their violence; they have an anger management problem.
- Abusive men are easy to identify. They are physically violent all of the time and to everyone.

Adapted from: Royal Australian College of General
Practitioners (1998) *Women and Violence*

2 What causes intimate partner violence?

In developing an understanding of intimate partner violence against women, the most central question for practitioners is that of causality. Are there identifiable sociological or psychological factors which can be reliably identified as contributing to, or even directly facilitating, some men's abuse of their female intimate partners? The question of causality is of core importance as the theories one adopts in answer to this question will colour one's practice interventions with women and with abusers and will influence wider social and legal sanctions. Kimmel (2002: 1333) notes that 'in recent years, a serious debate has erupted among activists, activist organizations, and individuals about the nature of domestic violence'. In this chapter, the principal contributions to this debate in the search for understandings of intimate partner violence will be reviewed. To facilitate as wide a review as possible of the issues under consideration, the material reviewed in this chapter will be drawn from sociological, psychological, and activist literature of both Western and, to a more limited extent, non-Western cultures.

Alternative approaches

Jasinski (2001: 5–16) distinguishes between micro-level theories, which seek to explain violence by looking at the socio-psychological or individual characteristics of either the abuser or the abused, and macro-level and socio-cultural theories, which focus on the social and cultural conditions which make violence likely. Kirkwood (1993: 13) suggests that while research in Britain in the 1960s and 70s tended to focus on a psychological approach to woman abuse, work in the USA tended to be sociologically focused. She makes a distinction between the 'traditional' perspectives, in which she includes the psychological and sociological approaches, and the 'feminist' perspective.

The 'traditional' approaches

The family conflict approach

The family violence perspective can be traced in large part to the work of Gelles (1974) and Straus (1977) in the 1970s when they developed quantitative methodologies to examine a variety of family violence issues. Gelles was the first, in 1974, to point to the high level of violence in American families. Straus, Gelles and Steinmetz (1980) conducted the first US national domestic violence survey in 1975 and a subsequent larger resurvey in 1985 (Straus and Gelles, 1990). They take the somewhat pessimistic view that with the exception of the police and the military in times of war, the family is society's most violent social institution (Gelles, 1993: 31–43). The findings from the 1975 survey (which surveyed only married and cohabiting couples) found a 16% overall rate of husband to wife abuse which included both minimum and severe forms of violence, and a 3.8% rate for severe violence. The greatest controversy within the emerging battered women's movement was generated by their finding that the rates of wife to husband violence were 11.6% for overall violence and 4.65% for severe violence. In their second and larger resurvey (Straus and Gelles, 1990), they reported that while there had been a reduction in the overall rate of violence in the home, with the husband to wife violence falling by 28%, the wife to husband violence dropped by only 4.3%. Consequently husbands were now more likely than wives to be victims of violence (12.1% as against 11.3% for women). The implications of this finding and the controversies to which it has given rise will be reviewed in greater detail in Chapter 3. The Conflict Tactics Scale (CTS) was originally developed by Straus and Gelles at the University of New Hampshire in the 1970s and used (in slightly differing forms) in their survey research. Firstly it is premised on the inevitability of conflict in human relationships and by extension the existence of conflict between all the configurations of family relationships.

In view of the sensitive nature of family violence and the perceived difficulty of getting a random population sample to reply to a questionnaire asking them about such private and potentially illegal acts, it is surprising that the 1985 survey achieved an 84% response rate. Straus acknowledges that the presentation of the instrument 'in the context of disagreements' was designed to facilitate and legitimise responses (1990: 5: 181–202). Presenting intimate partner violence as simply one way in which conflicts get resolved, decontextualised and devoid of any reference to either the motivation or consequences of these actions, has been one of the major criticisms of the CTS.

Dobash and Dobash (1992; 1998) have been amongst the loudest critics of the CTS and have drawn attention to a number of problems with the instrument. They point to the danger of combining forms of violence in a 'sum index' with the result that 'two slaps are counted the same as two knife attacks'. Currie (1998: 101) proposes that the problem with the CTS is that it is 'research rather than theory driven' with the result that even though Gelles and Straus (1988) themselves recognise that power and control are cited by both men and women research participants, these 'disappear from their interpretation of findings from the CTS' (Currie, 1998: 102).

Social stress as an explanation for violence

Within the family violence perspective, social stress is perhaps the explanation most commonly proposed by both professionals and the general public. Straus

(1990: 181–201) analysed the results of the 1985 National Family Violence survey to assess the extent to which social stress is associated with spousal violence. He found that the higher the stress score, the higher the rate of assault between spouses. However, the relationship is even more marked for wife to husband violence. While arguing that a major cause of violence in families is a high level of stress, he points out that most of the couples in the sample who were subject to high degrees of stress were not violent. This finding suggests that the relationship between stress and violence may not be causal and he concedes that his conclusions are 'not proved by the findings' (Straus, 1990: 199). Straus recognises that violence is only one of many possible responses to stress and suggests a number of mediating variables to explain his findings. These variables include exposure to violence in childhood, social support and approval of violence. The most important of these variables was approval of slapping a spouse, with a 456% difference in the rate of assault by husbands who approved of slapping their spouse.

Socio-economic factors such as low income, low educational achievement and criminality have also been perceived as variables in family violence statistics, both as causative factors in their own right and as the mediators between stress and violence (Heise and Garcia-Moreno, 2002: 99). While there is little consensus in the literature regarding the relationship between low educational achievement and higher levels of marital violence (Straus, 1990), some studies have identified a relationship between unemployment, low income and increased levels of violence (Vieraitis and Williams, 2002). Black *et al.* (1999), in a wide-ranging meta analysis of North American studies, found that low income, as distinct from employment status, presented consistently as a significant variable for intimate male partner violence.

In the Irish context, Watson and Parsons' (2005) national prevalence study explored the risk of severe abuse by the respondents' socio-economic status. They divided the occupations of the respondents into seven broad categories, based on their current or former form of employment or business): managerial and professional (e.g. company owners, doctors, teachers); technical and skilled trades (e.g. skilled manual occupations such as carpenters); self-employed (e.g. farmers and owners of small businesses); clerical (e.g. secretaries); services (e.g. shop assistants, waitresses); semi-skilled (e.g. drivers and machine operatives); routine (e.g. cleaners); and unknown. Their analysis showed that the lowest lifetime risk for both men and women was found amongst the managerial/professional and clerical groups while the highest risk for women was found amongst routine workers and women working in services or semi-skilled occupations (Watson and Parsons, 2005: 111). They point out, however, that these figures cannot be taken at face value, as these differences by socio-economic group are not statistically significant when other factors such as age, marital status and decision making within the relationship are controlled. Their analysis of the relationship between household income and risk of abuse further emphasises the complexity of the connection between socio-economic factors and intimate partner violence. In their analysis they found that while the highest risk for women was in the households with the lowest annual income, those in the highest income bracket had a level of risk almost as high, and much higher than for those in the second highest income bracket (Watson and Parsons, 2005: 112). This would appear to confirm Heise and Garcia-Moreno's (2002) contention that there are exceptions to the protection that higher income can offer to women, and intimate partner violence cuts across all socio-economic groups.

Social learning theory

In the public discourse, the 'cycle of violence' or the intergenerational transmission of violence, as it is more formally known, is possibly the most commonly accepted 'reason' for male violent behaviour within the home. Based on Bandura's (1973) social learning theory it proposes that the principal explanatory variable in the production of violence is the belief that people imitate or 'model' what they experience and see. Bandura (1973) pointed to the family, culture, subculture and the media as the primary sources in which violence is learned.

As with other theoretical explanations, social learning theory has been heavily criticised as inadequate. The work of Kaufman and Ziegler (1987) is often cited to disprove the proposition that the use of violence can be transmitted from one's family of origin. They found that the rate of intergenerational transmission of violence was 30%, which implies that the majority of those who witness or experience violence do not go on to perpetrate violence. However, a number of other studies can be cited which suggest that violence in one's family of origin can be a significant risk factor for the use of violence to one's adult intimate partner (Hotaling and Sugarman, 1986; Pagelow, 1984). More recent studies have continued to find a positive relationship. The Ellsberg *et al.* (1999) study in Nicaragua found that a history of violence in the husband's family was one of a number of factors that were significantly associated with his use of violence to his wife. The Black *et al.* (1999) meta review concluded that, even though the effects of adverse childhood experiences may be statistically small, they are consistently found as an increased risk marker for adult partner aggression.

Watson and Parsons' (2005: 118–119) Irish study also found a 'sharply increased risk' of experiencing abuse if a woman's father was abusive to her mother. They also found an increased risk where there was abuse in the partner's family of origin. They go on to stress, however, that abuse in the family of origin does not predetermine a pattern of abuse in an adult intimate relationship. They point out that the majority (70–75%) of those who were aware of abuse between their own parents or their partner's parents did not experience abuse themselves as adults. This figure reflects almost exactly the figure reported by Kaufman and Ziegler in 1987, cited above.

Recognising the lack of reliable empirical data to support or disapprove the inter-generational transmission of violence hypothesis, Heyman and Smith Slep (2002) utilised the data from the 1985 US Family Violence Survey to analyse a number of aspects of the hypothesis. With a data set of 6,002 participants, they examined the relationship between exposure to partner abuse in the family of origin and adult partner abuse perpetration or victimisation. As in the findings of Watson and Parsons (2005), they found that family of origin violence was associated with the perpetration of contemporary physical partner abuse, but also concluded that the cycle of violence is 'not a sealed fate'. The most typical outcome for those who had been exposed to family of origin violence, whether inter-parental or parent–child, or both, is to be non-violent in their adult relationships and families.

Learned helplessness

In the work of Lenore Walker (1979), a psychiatrist who has worked with hundreds of 'battered women', sociological theory and psychology begin to overlap and she has popularised the 'learned helplessness' theory. Walker (1993: 135) uses the term 'learned helplessness' to describe the psychological effects of living in an abusive relationship. She is at pains, however, to point out that it does 'not mean that women learn to behave in a helpless way'. This inherently contradictory terminology may have contributed to the many criticisms that her theory has provoked.

Walker's 1979 work, *The Battered Woman*, introduced to a wide readership the concept of the 'cycle of violence' (not to be confused with the intergenerational transmission of violence discussed above). From her study of hundreds of case histories she proposed that violent episodes between intimate partners are preceded by periods of mounting tension, and followed by a stage of apology and contrition in which the batterer tries to compensate for his violence by being especially caring. She suggests that it is this cycle of tension, violence and contrition which leads women to be passive (1979: 55–70). Here and in later work (1991; 1993), she introduced the concept of the Battered Woman Syndrome (BWS), which she described as 'a group of transient psychological symptoms that are frequently observed in a particular recognizable pattern in women who report having been physically, sexually and/or seriously psychologically abused' (1993: 135). She has developed a specific therapeutic intervention, 'survivor therapy', to treat women who may experience these transient symptoms as a result of abusive relationships. The symptoms of BWS are similar to those of post-traumatic stress disorder (PTSD) and the syndrome has been used successfully as a defence in court cases where women have been charged with murdering abusive partners. Walker, however, is aware of the risk of labels such as 'learned helplessness' and BWS in leading to the pathologising of women who may experience these effects of abuse.

In contrast, studies such as the influential review of 400 empirical studies by Hotaling and Sugarman (1990) found that there was no evidence that a woman's personality characteristics influence her chance of becoming a victim of wife assault. They identified variables such as her financial dependence, shame and fear of threats and retaliation as more likely predictive risk factors of violence.

Alcohol use and violence

The association of heavy drinking and wife beating amongst 'lower-class men' is a common stereotype that Kantor and Straus (1990: 203–224) describe as the 'drunken bum' theory. Hotaling and Sugarman, in their comprehensive analysis, found that alcohol abuse was a significant risk factor in wife abuse (1986: 111), and Black *et al.*, in their meta analysis (1999: 7), also report that in all the studies which have investigated this relationship, a significant association was found. Leonard's (1999) review in the same year also confirmed the association between alcoholism, or alcohol abuse, and domestic abuse. Fals-Stewart (2003) found in a clinical study that the odds that a husband would be physically violent to his wife on a day that he was drinking were increased 8–11 fold. Leonard and Quigley (1999) found in a community sample that alcohol use by a male partner was more likely to be present in episodes of severe or moderate violence as compared with incidents of verbal violence.

There is, however, a lack of consensus as to the mechanisms by which alcohol functions as a risk factor for abuse. As Leonard concluded, 'alcohol is neither a necessary nor a sufficient cause of marital aggression' (1999: 132). This is evidenced in the Irish Prevalence study (Watson and Parsons, 2005) which explored the role and effects of a number of 'potential triggers' on episodes of severe abuse. In response to the question as to whether alcohol was involved in these episodes, and if so, who had been drinking, they found that alcohol was involved 'some of the time' for 44% of respondents, 'all of the time' for 27% and 'never' for 29%. This suggests, as Watson and Parsons point out, that the results do not support a strong causal link between alcohol use and the perpetration of intimate partner violence. For those for whom alcohol was a factor, they found that in over 90% of cases it was either the abuser or both partners who were drinking at the time of an assault.

A number of studies have attempted to disentangle this complex relationship between alcohol use and partner violence. Testa *et al.* (2003) explored the degree of severity of physical violence when the perpetrator was intoxicated in a small sample of newly weds. Their principal finding was that violent episodes in which the husband had been drinking were more severe than episodes in which there was no drink involved (Testa *et al.*, 2003: 740). They also found, however (to their apparent surprise), that there were discrepancies between the husbands' and the wives' reports regarding the levels of violence. As they found, no relationship between the level of wives' tendency to 'underreport violence, particularly severe violence', and their consumption of alcohol, they believe that a 'more plausible explanation' involves the men's underreporting of violence, 'particularly of severe violence' (Testa *et al.*, 2003: 740). This finding is consistent with the work of Dobash and Dobash (2004) and the analysis of the dynamics of intimate partner violence developed by the Duluth Intervention Project (Pence and Paymar, 1993) which includes the denial and minimisation of violence by abusive partners in their well-known Power and Control Wheel. This was discussed in Chapter 1.

Kantor and Straus (1990) explored the relationship between alcohol use, socio-economic status, beliefs about wife beating and actual rates of violence. They found that while there was a clear linear association between heavy drinking and abuse, they point out that 'it is extremely important not to overlook the substantial amount of wife abuse by abstainers and moderate drinkers' (Kantor and Straus, 1990: 211). They also found that in 76% of violent episodes, alcohol was not used immediately prior to the assault. As in other studies (which will be discussed in greater detail below) they found that men who held traditional views regarding the legitimacy of slapping their wife were more likely to have used violence in the previous twelve months. They make clear that it is the combination of economic status, approval of wife abuse and drinking that increases the likelihood of partner violence, but that the causal mechanisms of these factors are not elucidated by the data. Heise (1998: 273) suggests that alcohol use may contribute to family violence by providing a topic for arguments, while also recognising that feminists have been somewhat wary of acknowledging that alcohol plays any role in the aetiology of abuse as it may be used as an excuse for this behaviour.

In a study by Livingston (2011), it was found that there was a clear relationship between alcohol outlet density and domestic violence. The more opportunities there are to buy alcohol, the more likely that severe domestic violence will occur. In a study involving 13 countries by Graham *et al.* (2011) as part of the GENACIS study (Gender, Alcohol, and Culture: An International Study), it was also found that severity ratings were significantly higher for incidents in which one or both partners had been drinking compared to incidents in which neither partner had been drinking. They suggest that alcohol reduces cognitive abilities and impairs problem solving. Alcohol also increases risk taking and reduces awareness of the consequences of one's actions. Despite cultural differences between these diverse countries (European, African and Latin American countries, the USA and India) the findings of this study were consistent. There was greater aggression associated with alcohol abuse at the time of the assault. While these studies highlight that alcohol will increase levels of abuse and aggression, they do not provide a reason as to why these incidents occur between men and women.

Feminist analysis of violence against women

Stark, (2007: 28) cites the Women's Advocates Shelter in St. Paul, Minnesota in 1974, and Dobash and Dobash (1992: 25) cite the Chiswick refuge in London in 1971, as examples of how emergency housing projects for battered women arose from women coming together in consciousness raising groups. For the activists 'battering was an integral part of women's oppression; women's liberation its solution' (Schechter, 1982: 34).

Dobash and Dobash (1992: 25) also trace the origins of the battered women's movement directly to the wider feminist movement and contend that 'most of the early shelter groups arose out of women's liberation consciousness raising groups'. They place these developments within the radical feminist tradition of feminist thought suggesting that the 'pro-woman' orientation of that tradition 'has led to a concentration on the central importance of gender, the intimate domination of women under patriarchy and a consideration of its institutional and ideological forms' (Dobash and Dobash, 1992: 75).

Concern about violence against women and the quest to understand its cause(s) can, however, be found in much earlier traditions of feminist thinking. In an article published in the *Contemporary Review* in 1878 (the period usually described as the 'first wave' of feminism, i.e. late nineteenth to early twentieth centuries), British journalist Frances Cobbe describes (in sometimes graphic detail) the serious assaults that women experienced in all social classes of contemporary British society. She goes on to ask why this 'persistent torture of women' is tolerated and concludes that:

> The notion that a man's wife is his PROPERTY, in the sense in which a horse is his property . . . every brutal minded man, and many a man who in other relations of life is not brutal, entertains more or less vaguely the notion that his wife is his thing, and is ready to ask with indignation (as we read again and again in the police reports), of any one who interferes with his treatment of her, 'May I not do what I will with my own?'
>
> (Cobbe, 1878: 62)

In these succinct lines, a nineteenth-century journalist and activist identifies what has become the key concept in the modern feminist approach to intimate partner violence, namely the power differential between women and men, which is understood by the latter as proprietorship and control, and experienced by the former as submission.

The roots of these concepts of ownership and control of women are to be found in the cultural mechanisms which give expression to society's beliefs and values – namely the legal and religious structures and discourses which determine the distribution of power at micro-individual and macro-societal levels. Feminist analysis proposes that patriarchy is the social and cultural mechanism which both expresses and reinforces violence against women.

Patriarchy has been defined as 'a system of society, government etc. ruled by a man and with descent through the male line' (*Oxford Modern English Dictionary*, 1995: 784).

Religious influences

O'Faolain and Martines (1973), in their work *Not in God's Image*, trace the cultural position of women in Western Civilisation from the time of the ancient Greeks. Their fascinating and revealing quotations from secular and religious literature paint a comprehensive picture of Western society's patriarchal attitudes to women over two millennia. They begin their historical odyssey with Athenian men who knew how to manage the females in their world: 'Mistresses we keep for pleasure, concubines for daily attendance upon our person and wives to bear us legitimate children and be our faithful housekeepers' (Demosthenes, 3rd-century BC, cited in O'Faolain and Martines, 1973). Despite their many differences, both Islamic and Judeo Christian traditions agree on the place of women in the eyes of their all male God: 'Men are superior to women on account of the qualities with which God hath gifted the one above the other, and on account of the outlay they make from their substance for them' (Sura 4, verse 38, *Koran*: trans. Rodwell, 1977). St Paul was probably the most influential apostolic writer in moulding the early Christian theological understanding of the roles of women and men with exhortations such as 'The head of the woman is the man . . . forasmuch as he is the image and the glory of God: but the woman is the glory of the man' (1 Corinthians, 11: 3, 7–9). This theme is picked up again and again throughout church history. The following quotation from the twelfth-century AD Gratian, is one of many cited by O'Faolain and Martines (1973: 130):

> Women should be subject to their men. The natural order for mankind is that women should serve men and children their parents, for it is just that the lesser serve the greater. . . . Women's authority is nil; let her in all things be subject to the rule of man. . . . And neither can she teach, nor be a witness, nor give a guarantee, nor sit in judgement.
>
> *(Corpus Iuris Canonici)*

Later recent religious leaders such as Martin Luther in 1531 (Luther, trans.Tappert, 1967) and John Knox (1558) defended this patriarchal tradition. Luther, for example, expounded on women's natural inferiority to men and proposed that 'Women ought to stay at home; the way they were created indicates this, for they have broad hips and a fundament to sit upon, keep house, and bear children' (cited in Dobash and Dobash, 1979: 53). Knox (1558) put his views somewhat more succinctly, when he wrote that 'woman in her greatest perfection was made to serve and obey man'.

Western secular influences

The great secular thinkers of the Western philosophical tradition were no less certain of women's place in society and no less intent on keeping them there. Writing about the emerging debate on the education of women, Rousseau (1762) proposed:

> Thus women's entire education should be planned in relation to men. To please men, to be useful to them, to win their love and respect, to raise them as children, care for them as adults, counsel and console them, make their lives sweet and pleasant: these are women's duties in all ages and these are what they should be taught from childhood on.
>
> (Rousseau, 1762: 455)

Patriarchy and the family

In view of these cultural and religious understandings of the dominating relationship of men over women, it is to be expected that marriage in its varying legal and social manifestations would reflect these values. St. Paul expresses it simply: 'Wives, submit yourself unto your own husbands, as unto the Lord. For the husband is the head of the wife' (Ephesians 5: 22–23). The expression 'to take one's hand in marriage' comes directly from the ancient Roman (Latin) phrase *in manu*, where *Manus* meant the power exercised by the head of the family over his wife and children (O'Faolain and Martines, 1973: 41).

Martin (1981), in her work *Battered Wives*, traces the patriarchal tradition in the development of the modern family. Recognising that 'The historical roots of our patriarchal family models are ancient and deep' (Martin, 1981: 25), she outlines the way in which this family form became the means by which men control and dominate their female partners. 'With the advent of the pairing marriage, the man seized the reins in the home and began viewing the people in it as units of property that comprised his wealth – in short, as chattel.' The word 'family' is derived from the Roman word *familia*, signifying the totality of slaves belonging to an individual. The slave owner had absolute power of life and death over the human beings who 'belonged to him' (Martin, 1981: 27).

One can rarely find a text which explores the feminist analysis of intimate partner violence that does not refer to the 'landmark statement of this approach' namely Dobash and Dobash's (1979) *Violence Against Wives: A Case Against the Patriarchy*. In this important work, Dobash and Dobash trace the role of women and the power of their husbands in Western legal, religious and political history since earliest Roman times to show that violence against women is 'the extension of the domination and control of husbands over their wives' (1979: 15) and how this control is socially constructed. They suggest that legal, historical, literary and religious writings all contribute to an understanding of the unique status of women, which composes the kernel of the explanation of why it is women who have become the 'appropriate' victims of marital violence (Dobash and Dobash, 1979: 32).

Rebutting the traditional explanations and justifications for this violence, they draw on a wide repertoire of historical material to show how patriarchy was justified and maintained in each historical epoch. In early Roman society, (from which much of Western society's legal and cultural traditions have evolved), the family was one of strongest patriarchies known, presided over by a male head, who was priest, magistrate and owner of all material and human properties and had absolute power over everything and everyone (Dobash and Dobash, 1979: 34). Within this system, a woman had few, if any, alternatives outside of marriage, and was her husband's property within it. Husbands and fathers could put a woman to death without recourse to public trial, and it seems reasonable to assume that these statutes reflected the general acceptance of physical abuse of women and legitimised their subjection through force.

Dobash and Dobash trace these traditions of power and subjugation through the Middle Ages, through the rise of the state and the power of the king when the ideology supported the patriarchal form of authority in the nuclear family and 'equated loyalty to the patriarch with allegiance to the monarch and to God' (1979: 49). These unequal power relations continued through the rise of Protestantism and capitalism.

They show how legal statutes buttressed these ideologies. 'Matrimony deprived a woman of her legal rights, set different standards for her behaviour, and gave her husband the legal right to inflict corporal punishment upon her' (Dobash and Dobash, 1979: 60). In English law (which influenced American law and Irish law), a woman, on getting married, surrendered her legal identity, her rights to own property, to personal credit and to the guardianship of any children she might have:

> The wife came under the control of her husband and he had the legal right to use force against her in order to ensure that she fulfilled her wifely obligations, which included consummation of the marriage, co-habitation, maintenance of conjugal rights, sexual fidelity and general obedience and respect for his wishes.
>
> (Dobash and Dobash, 1979: 60)

An Irish experience

The deceased Irish writer John McGahern's autobiography provides a fascinating and dispassionate account of the operation of this ideology within an Irish family in the early part of the twentieth-century. In his *Memoir* (2005) McGahern describes, without comment, the consistent cruelty and strategies of control which his father utilised towards all of his children. While he does not recount his father using physical violence towards his first wife (John's mother, who died when he was a young child), his accounts of his father's expectations of his wife and his neglect of her during her final illness, provides an illuminating and dispassionate description of the patriarchal expectations of a traditional Irish Catholic man of the time. The following extracts describe, in McGahern's understated way, the influence of a cruel and controlling father and husband:

> I felt the same fear when my father was in the house. There was always tension when he was in the house, scolding over how money was being wasted, or the poor way the house was being run, or my mother's relatives. In certain moods he did not need a reason to fall into a passion of complaint, which then fed off his own anger.
>
> (McGahern, 2005: 22)

> My father would come down the stairs in his shirt and trousers and unlaced boots. The fire had to be going by then, the kettle boiling. We went through these mornings on tiptoe... The house went completely quiet while he shaved. Sometimes he would nick himself with the razor and we'd bring him bits of newspaper to staunch the bleeding. A clean dry towel had to be placed in his hands as soon as he washed ... Then he would sit down to breakfast, facing the big sideboard mirror. At this time Bridgie McGovern [housemaid/ nanny] would have served him, later my sisters. He never acknowledged the server or any of the small acts of service, but would erupt into complaint if there was a fault – a knife or dish or fork or spoon missing, or something accidentally spilled or dropped.
>
> (McGahern, 2005: 32–33)

These accounts of the daily details of McGahern's childhood provide a glimpse into the unremarkable exercise of expected patriarchal privilege in an ordinary family.

Patriarchy and violence

Within the feminist perspective of intimate partner violence the socio-cultural context shapes, fosters, and encourages the use of violence to maintain inequitable power relationships in all areas of women's lives, but especially in the home (Marin and Russo, 1999). O'Faolain and Martines (1973) again provide numerous examples of explicit permission and even exhortations to husbands to use physical violence against their wives. The following is from *The Rules of Marriage* compiled by Friar Cherubino of Siena in the mid fifteenth-century:

> You should beat her I say only when she commits a serious wrong; for example, if she blasphemes against God or a saint, if she mutters the devil's name, if she likes being at the window and lends a ready ear to dishonest young men, or if she has taken to bad habits or bad company, or commits some other wrong that is a mortal sin. Then readily beat her, not in rage but out of charity and concern for her soul, so that the beating will redound to your merit and her good.
>
> (Cited in O'Faolain and Martines, 1973: 177)

Common proverbs from around the world also provide an insight into the manner in which violence has been seen as a legitimate means of enforcing male privilege and control over women.

- 'As both a good horse and a bad horse heed the spur, so both a good woman and a bad woman need the stick.' (From Italy.)
- 'A bride received into the home is like a horse that you have just bought; you break her in by continually mounting her and continually beating her.' (From China.)
- 'Love well, whip well.' (Benjamin Franklin.)
- 'A spaniel, a woman and a walnut tree, the more they're beaten the better they be.' (From England.)

(All cited in Grant, 1999: 164)

These proverbs expose the cross cultural extent of the old Roman concept of patriarchy, which, as was seen in a previous section, involved the ownership of women, children, slaves and animals, even in societies not directly influenced by Roman civilisation and culture.

The legal benchmark for violence

While the first legal rejection of the right to 'chastisement' occurred in England in 1829 (Dobash and Dobash, 1979: 63) the following can still be found in court reports over ten years later. In 1840, in the case of Cecilia Maria Cochrane, who ran away from her husband, the judge of the Queen's Bench stated in his judgement:

There can be no doubt of the general dominion which the law of England attributes to the husband over the wife; in Bacon, Abridgment, title 'Baron and Feme', it is stated thus: 'the husband hath by law power and dominion over his wife, and may keep her by force, within the bounds of duty, and may beat her, but not in a violent or cruel manner . . .'

(Dowling, 1841: 630)

Again in 1915, a London magistrate was still able to make the now infamous judgement that 'the husband of a nagging wife . . . could beat her at home provided the stick he used was no thicker than a man's thumb' (cited in Dobash and Dobash, 1979: 74).

Dobash and Dobash (1979) summarise their review of the legal, political, and economic institutions which reinforced patriarchal structures and ideology, suggesting it would have been inconceivable for them to have supported any other form of family relations. 'These ideals and their accompanying practices formed the foundations of the subordination and control of women' (Dobash and Dobash, 1979: 74).

Patriarchy in practice

The feminist perspective faces two challenges to its usefulness as an explanatory construct for intimate partner violence. Firstly, it must be possible to show that violence against intimate female partners correlates positively with other structural indicators of patriarchal social organisation, and secondly, the mechanism(s) by which patriarchal beliefs are mediated in individual relationships must be elucidated and demonstrable.

Vieraitis and Williams (2002) reviewed 14 studies that examined the relationship between gender equality and various forms of violence against women (including homicide). Gender equality was measured using 'economic, educational and occupational variables from the 1990 *Census of Population: Social and Economic Characteristics*' (Vieraitis and Williams, 2002: 46). While the findings of these studies were not entirely consistent, it was strongly evident that there was a relationship between women's inequality and rates of female homicide, rape and wife beating. These findings suggest that simple structural reforms of the position of women by reducing levels of inequality in the economic and political spheres, do not of themselves reduce violence against women. The mediating factors of attitudes and marital power dynamics may continue to 'contaminate' the marital relationship with patriarchal values of control and dominance.

Yllo's (1984) study throws light on these points. This study assessed marital equality on the basis of the relative decision making power of the husband and wife and related this to the use of violence. She found that the rate of wife-beating in couples where the husband is dominant is 50% higher than for wife dominant couples and more than 300% greater than for egalitarian couples. Commenting on the apparently contradictory finding that violence is higher where the wife is dominant than for egalitarian couples, she suggests that 'Evidently, wife dominance in decision making is met with physical aggression by some husbands . . . It appears that for many of these husbands, exercise of control in marriage requires resorting to the use of severe violence against their wives' (Yllo, 1984: 314–315).

In Watson and Parsons' (2005) Irish prevalence study, a similar relationship was found between decision making and a risk of violence. In cohabiting relationships the odds of a woman being severely abused are increased seven times where her partner makes decisions about household money, in comparison to couples where such decisions are made jointly. Where the woman makes the decisions about money, the chances of abuse are also increased, but to a lesser extent. These findings suggest that more than twenty years later, Yllo's (1984) analysis is still valid.

Beliefs about marital violence

The feminist perspective on intimate partner violence can also be interrogated by analysing the relationship between holding patriarchal beliefs and attitudes and either using, or supporting the use of, violence against female partners. A number of studies from both Western (e.g. Australia, Britain and the USA) and non-Western (e.g. Israel, Palestinian territories, and South Asian immigrant) societies have strongly supported a positive correlation between patriarchal attitudes and intimate partner violence. James *et al.* (2002), in a study of 130 voluntary attendees at a domestic violence perpetrator programme in Sydney, sought to elicit how these men constructed their use of violence to their intimate partners. They postulate two categories of forms of violence – 'tyrant' and 'exploder' violence. While as the name suggests:

> 'tyrants' used aggression, intimidation, verbal abuse and physical assault to assert domination and control over their partners . . . these men knew what they were doing and they intended to frighten, intimidate and punish. . . . The violence of 'exploders' in the study was sudden and explosive . . . and most often occurred in response to their partner's criticism.
>
> (James *et al.*, 2002: 4–5)

However, despite these differences the authors are clear that 'Explosive- and tyrant-type violence are not mutually exclusive but instead can be understood as on a continuum with men experiencing or reporting varying degrees of control and intentionality. From the woman's perspective, however, the outcome is the same' (James *et al.*, 2002: 6). Finding that most of the men came from traditional family models, where the father was the breadwinner and seen as 'the boss', they conclude that 'traditionally gendered roles are not surprising, but in the context of men's domestic violence they become the structural bedrock from which boys develop a sense of their own entitlement in relation to women as partners and mothers' (James *et al.*, 2002: 16).

In Hearn's 1998 UK study, he also analyses men's narratives regarding their use of violence to known women, suggesting that they can be characterised as denials, excuses or justifications (though he points out that these are not always discrete types of accounts) (Hearn, 1998: 144). He concludes that:

Men's accounts and explanations of violence take place in the context of men's power and generally reflect, indeed, reproduce, [*Hearn's emphasis*] these power relations. Not only may acts of violence be understood in terms of power and control, but so too may accounts and explanations given by men in interviews, conversations and other forms of talk. Men's accounts of violence are themselves usually within and examples of patriarchal domination and male domination.

Some of the examples he quotes from his study stunningly illustrate his conclusion e.g.:

> I wasn't violent to anyone. Except her. In all my life. I don't know why. I don't feel motivated towards violence towards anyone else. I think it were a feeling that I owned her. I owned this particular person and she were my property . . .
>
> (Hearn, 1998: 127)

Wood's (2004) qualitative study involving 22 inmates of a medium security prison in the USA, also explored the relationship between beliefs about gender relationships and the use of violence against female intimate partners. Her findings expose the complexity of social norms and the men's ability to hold two apparently contradictory codes of manhood at the same time. She found that all 22 of the participants believed that physically abusing their wives or girlfriends was 'a legitimate response to being disrespected as a man' (Wood, 2004: 562). A second theme which was closely related to the first was that a man is entitled to use violence to control or discipline 'his woman' (Wood, 2004: 563). One 23-year-old participant described this in a way which is startlingly similar to the proverbs quoted above. 'A woman's kind like a dog. You got to break 'em. A dog don't do right, you beat it 'til it do what you say. It either leave or be broke. Same with women.' A minority of the participants also expressed remorse and disassociation from 'really abusive men', while at the same time, expressing beliefs about their right to be respected and obeyed. Wood notes that 'all of the men alluded to what may be termed a "patriarchal" view of manhood which holds that men are superior to women', and are 'entitled to sex and other attention from their wives and girlfriends' (Wood, 2004: 568).

While holding to these 'US cultural narratives of masculinity', some also justified their violence on their feelings of not being 'real men' and personally embodying this ideal of manhood (Wood, 2004: 569).

These responses demonstrate the complexity of the social learning theory explanations of marital violence (discussed above). While many of the men referred to the way they were brought up, others recounted that 'my mama always taught me you're not supposed to put your hands on a woman' (Wood, 2004: 569). Thirteen of the participants held this latter chivalrous view of manhood, which requires men to respect and take care of women, but this view did not prevent them from severely abusing the women with whom they were intimate. Exploring this contradiction, Wood suggests that while they may subscribe to the cultural code of chivalry in an abstract way, they do not always relate it to their relationships with their intimate partners. They are in fact more likely to relate it to 'other women', such as mothers and daughters (Wood, 2004: 570). The ability to make such distinctions between 'other women' and their wives or girlfriends, is strongly suggestive of the strength of the dominant patriarchal view of intimate partners, which encourages control and dominance and permits the use of violence to achieve such control.

Non-Western cultures

Studies from non-Western societies have found similar patterns in the connection between patriarchal attitudes and partner abuse. In his work with Arab populations in the Palestinian West Bank and in Israel, Haj-Yahia (1998; 2003) suggests that:

> men's tendency to justify wife beating, blame wives for violence against them, and to some extent also hold violent husbands responsible for their behaviour are best explained by their non-egalitarian expectations of marriage, traditional attitudes towards women, and patriarchal beliefs about family life.
> (Haj-Yahia, 2003: 194)

In his 2003 study of 500 randomly chosen couples, he used a number of Attitude Inventory Scales to test the hypothesis that attitudes towards women, sex-role stereotypes, sexual conservatism, religiosity, familial patriarchal beliefs and marital role expectations would correlate significantly with a justification of wife beating, blaming women themselves for violence against them and not holding abusive and violent husbands responsible for their behaviour. His results supported this hypothesis and he argues that 'The results obtained . . . can be attributed to the patriarchal orientation of Arab culture on issues related to family life, marital relations, and gender roles in the family and society at large' (Haj-Yahia, 2003: 203). He concludes that his findings are highly consistent with the contention that the approval of wife beating and lenient treatment of [domestically] violent men are 'manifestations of patriarchy' (Haj-Yahia, 2003: 203).

Even though it is men who benefit from patriarchal gender norms, both men and women can subscribe to and support such norms within their families and communities. In a study which the authors believe is the first of its kind, Ahmad *et al.* (2004) explored the relationship between patriarchal beliefs amongst South Asian immigrant women (i.e. from India, Pakistan or Sri Lanka) in Canada. Using a telephone sample of 47 women who agreed to participate, they found that the experience of physical abuse in their intimate relationships in the previous five years, at 24%, was three times higher than the Canadian national prevalence figures of 8% (Ahmad *et al.*, 2004: 277). Their hypothesis was that a woman who held stronger patriarchal beliefs would be less likely to perceive a woman who had been assaulted by her husband as a victim of wife abuse. Using a series of questions to ascertain the level of acceptance of patriarchal norms amongst the sample (e.g. questions such as the acceptability of a man deciding whether his wife could work outside the home), and a vignette about a marital argument which resulted in injury to the woman, this hypothesis was supported. They point out that these findings are of importance because a woman's perception of abuse is likely to affect her helpseeking responses to such abuse, and also the likelihood of her offering help and support to another woman experiencing abuse.

In a study carried out in Ethiopia (Allen and Ni Raghallaigh, in press) based on qualitative focus groups in both urban and rural areas with a range of women of differing ages, the patriarchal beliefs within the culture were clearly visible. While various causes for violence against women were suggested, three were particularly prominent. The women mentioned poverty, lack of education and lack of equality as reasons for the violence that occurred. One participant stated the following as a cause of violence against women: 'The attitude of the community which doesn't consider the woman to be fully human'. Another made reference to the roles attributed to women and the lack of respect for these roles: 'Violence is because they are females. This is because of her sex, she has to be pregnant, to lactate and take care of children and in this process she did not get respect for this'. Some simply suggested that one received less recognition for being a woman and as a result women could be demeaned. According to one participant, this started at birth: 'The problem starts at home with the mother and family. We have different expectations for boys and girls. When we give birth, we acclaim the birth of boys five times, for girls only three times'. Such distinctions, from the time of one's birth, continue on throughout a woman's life, exposing her to being a lesser person, a lesser citizen and therefore amenable to domestic violence.

From values to violence

Whilst these studies strongly support the feminist analysis that traditional patriarchal beliefs and attitudes to women provide a context and support for violence, this analysis must also demonstrate the mechanism(s) by which these attitudes influence the intimate relationship. Birns *et al.* (1994) have examined the sex-role socialisation of women and men as contributory factors in this power imbalance because, they suggest, 'central to understanding men's abuse of their partners is the use of such constructs as entitlement and sex-roles'. Identifying that 'men's expectations that their wives will treat them as members of the dominant class (i.e. will serve, listen to, and "obey" them)', they highlight the roles of parents, teachers, peers and wider social networks, in shaping gender-based differences in conflict resolution strategies. These gendered differential patterns in speaking and responding to male and female children result in a 'tendency for males to use aggressive strategies, both as children and as adults', while 'females learn to be deferential'. They conclude that 'this gendered process of socialization mirrors the dynamics of battering relationships', as they both reflect and contribute to power disparities in male/female relationships (Birns *et al.*, 1994: 57).

Hyden (1994) studied 141 Swedish couples, in order to explore the social psychological process of woman battering in marriage from the perspectives of the male perpetrator, the female victim and the couple engaged in the joint project of marriage (Hyden, 1994: vii). For the purposes of her analysis of 'woman battering as a marital act' she separates the act into three phases: the pre-history of the violent act, the violent incident, and the aftermath. She concluded:

> that the role of the pre-history was constitutive in producing a hierarchical organization within the marital project, following a *basic pattern of dominance and subordination* . . . Due to the fact that the pre-history of the violence turns into the violent phase itself, the hierarchical pattern becomes transfixed in a single image: the man in the dominant position and the woman in the subordinate position . . . During the violent incident, the hierarchical organization within the marriage assumes a more definite shape. By the use of violence, the man usurps power over the woman. 'Power over' refers to domination and control.
>
> (Hyden, 1994: 159–161)

As Stark (2007), in his study of coercive control points out, women in most societies have made considerable gains in legal representation and public participation. But:

> Men had no need for coercive control as long as women's daily regime of obedience was fully regulated by religion, and custom or sexism was codified in the law . . . its deployment today is designed to stifle and co-opt women's gains; foreclose negotiation over the organization, extent and substance of women's activities in and around the home; obstruct their access to support; close the spaces in which they can critically on their lives; and reimpose obsolete forms of dependence and personal service by micromanaging the enactment of stereotypic gender roles through 'sexism with a vengeance'.
>
> (Stark, 2007: 194)

Conclusion

This chapter has explored the reasons for the abuse of women. Does the cause of domestic violence lie in individual characteristics, in families' circumstances or in the cultures in which they are located? It has reviewed international literature which has either supported or challenged understandings of domestic violence which have been variously titled 'micro-level', 'traditional' or 'family violence' approaches. These have included the family conflict research undertaken primarily in the USA as well as the contributions of exchange theory which places the root of violence within the imbalances of resources in individual family units. The complex issue of the intergenerational transmission of violence and the controversial contribution of Walker's (1979; 1984; 1993) learned helplessness and Battered Woman Syndrome in the treatment of battered women and the defence of those who kill their abusers, have also been reviewed. Research into the role of stress, including socio-economic status and alcohol use has been outlined. This chapter has also provided an overview of what has become known as the feminist analysis of violence against women. The central concerns of such an analysis are male power and women's subservience rooted in social, religious and economically oppressive structures (Kelly, 2005; Dobash and Dobash, 1979), which are in turn supported by patriarchal norms and beliefs. These beliefs have been shown to justify the use of violence towards intimates, even within a wider cultural code of respect for women. The deep roots of these patriarchal beliefs both historically and transculturally have been illustrated by the breadth of material from a range of diverse sources.

It could be accepted at this point that the feminist analysis as outlined above provides a comprehensive and adequate explanation for the enduring social phenomenon that is domestic violence.

3 Gender symmetry and the process of leaving abusive relationships

The previous chapter has reviewed the principal contributions to the diverse approaches to understanding the causality of intimate partner violence. However, the debates surrounding domestic violence have not been limited to the issue of causality. Rather than reaching a consensus, the debates surrounding aetiology have now merged with the more recent controversies surrounding gender symmetry and directionality. The contention that women are also violent towards their male intimate partners has added even greater complexity to research and public policy in this area. In view of the importance of these more recent debates surrounding the understanding of intimate partner violence, this chapter will review the background and contrasting contributions within the literature to the issue of gender symmetry. It is important for practitioners working with abused women and men to understand these important differences, because in not understanding these distinctions, practitioners can be misled into thinking that women can be and are as violent as their male partners. It is important to understand the differences between these two forms of violence as confusing one with the other will lead practitioners to make unhelpful interventions.

Gender symmetry: are women as violent as men?

Sexual (or gender) symmetry has become one of the most hotly debated topics in the area of intimate partner violence theory building and in many ways reflects the feminist versus family violence divide referred to in the previous chapter (e.g. Straus and Gelles, 1990; Steinmetz, 1977/78; Dobash and Dobash, 1992; Straus, 1977, 1980, 1990; Saunders, 2002; and Kimmel, 2002). The debate, however, has not remained in the realm of academia, but has influenced social policy decision making and media comment (Allen and Forgey, 2007).

The gender neutral view of intimate partner violence, which Dobash and Dobash (1992) describe as counterintuitive and counterfactual, is indicative of the popularised application of studies which suggest that women are as violent, or even more prone to violence, than men (Steinmetz, 1977/78; Stets and Straus, 1990; Archer, 2000). As discussed in the previous chapter, Straus et al. (1980), and Stets and Straus (1990), using the data from the National Family Violence (NFV) survey, found that while 12.1% of wives were victims of their husbands' violence in the year prior to the 1975 survey, 11.6% of husbands were victims of their wives' violence. In the 1985 NFV survey these figures had changed to 11.3% of wives and 12.1% of husbands being victims of violence. This prompted Stets and Straus (1990: 227) to comment that the marriage licence is 'a hitting licence' and that the rates of perpetrating spousal violence were higher for wives than for husbands. Using the NFV survey and related data as 'fuel', Steinmetz (1977/78) ignited the symmetry debate by proposing the existence of the 'battered husband syndrome'. In her paper of this title, she quotes a number of studies which she claims found that rates of violence by men and women were either 'identical' or 'very similar' or the violence of wives 'exceeds that of husbands' (Steinmetz, 1977–78: 499–503). In reply this was met with charges of 'the battered data syndrome' (Pleck *et al.*, 1977–78) in which the data on which Steinmetz-based her conclusions was re-examined and her analysis severely criticised. For example, Pleck *et al.* (1977–78: 680) state quite bluntly that 'a summary statement that the percentage of wives having used physical violence "often exceeds" that of husbands is incorrect and even irresponsible'.

These claims were challenged in an almost forensically detailed fashion in papers by Saunders (1988) and Schwartz and DeKeseredy (1993). In his critique Saunders takes issue with the homicide figures quoted by McNeely and Robinson-Simpson (1987), and like Pleck *et al.* (1977–78: 179), he accuses Steinmetz and McNeely and Robinson-Simpson of being 'selective with the data they presented'.

The second NFV survey (Stets and Straus, 1990: 151–165) finding that 'women assault their partners at about the same rate as men' and that they may even be more likely to initiate violence than their partners, accentuated the debate, and again both the data and methodology have been rigorously critiqued. The primary target of these critiques has been the reliability of the Conflict Tactics Scale. Stets and Straus (1990: 162) proffer an explanation for their controversial findings by suggesting that (1) battered women may incorporate violence in their own behavioural repertory; (2) they may adopt the norm of reciprocal violence; and (3) the use of violence in one sphere, such as child care, may carry over into their marital relationship. Their findings do, however, show that women are more likely to use less severe violence than their male partners, and that women are more likely to sustain more serious injury requiring more medical care and sick leave. Intriguingly, they attempt to explain away this latter point by suggesting that women may find it easier to adopt the 'sick role' as they have fewer work and time constraints than men.

Schwartz and DeKeseredy (1993: 250), in their paper on the construction of the 'typical' abused woman, trace the shifts and turns in Straus and Gelles' position on female to male violence, 'whose dozens of articles and books have at times contradicted their other articles and books'. Given the latters' 'status' as the 'standard canon in the field', they point to the danger of using the NFV survey data to cast doubt on the self-defence thesis of female to male violence and Straus and Gelles' justification for drawing attention to the issue of female violence 'because even minor violence by wives greatly increases the risk of subsequent severe assault by the husband' (Straus and Gelles, 1990: 120).

Critiques of gender symmetry: the new millennium

As the debate continues into this millennium, Kimmel (2002) and Saunders (2002) have reviewed a range of studies which have followed on the work of Straus and Gelles, Stets and Steinmetz, and which claim to replicate their findings of sexual symmetry. Kimmel focuses particularly on the meta analysis by Archer (2000) and review by Fiebert (1998) which cite 100 empirical studies which suggest equivalent rates of violence for both sexes. Having reviewed the methodology of all of the 76 studies and 16 literature reviews, (including one study which used comic strips from 1950 as evidence of wives' greater aggression), Kimmel (2002: 1336) concludes that Fiebert's 'scholarly annotated bibliography thus turns out to be far more of an ideological polemic than a serious scholarly undertaking'. Both he and Saunders (2002) compare the data found in US Crime Victimization studies with the family violence studies which use the Conflict Tactics Scale (CTS) and support the gender symmetry thesis. The former, unlike the CTS-based studies, include sexual assaults, ask about assaults by ex-spouses or ex-partners, and tend to have larger sample sizes (usually national or state wide). They uniformly find gender asymmetry in rates of domestic violence. One of these large scale victimisation studies, the 1998 National Violence Against Women survey, found that men physically assaulted their partners at three times the rate at which women assaulted their partners (Tjaden and Thoennes, 2000).

Saunders, in his paper 'Are Physical Assaults by Wives and Girlfriends a Major Social Problem?' notes three limitations of the Archer (2000) and Fiebert (1998) reviews: (1) they fail to include the motives of each partner; (2) they ignore the rates of initiation of violence by each partner and in particular episodes; (3) they ignore the physical and psychological consequences of the violence to each partner (Saunders, 2002: 1429). Saunders (2002) pays particular attention to the homicide rates in the USA for both sexes, pointing out that 70% of all partner homicides in the past few years were women killed by their male partners while 30% were males killed by their female partners, and that the homicide figures prior to the mid 1980s were far more gender equal. Kimmel (2002) in his paper credits this unparalleled decline in male homicide rates by female intimates to the provision of shelters and helplines for battered women. He quotes an explanation by Professor of Criminal Justice, James Alan Fox, that 'because more battered women have escape routes, fewer wife batterers are being killed' (Kimmel, 2002: 1355). In situations where men or women are killed by their partners, Saunders (2002) asserts that studies show that the use of violence in self-defence is estimated to be 7–10 times less frequent for husbands than for wives.

Comparing differing methodologies

As one of the criticisms of the CTS methodology is that closed questions do not give any understanding of the motivations and consequences of the reported violence, Currie (1998) takes on the challenge of elucidating the meaning of such quantitative research findings for both female and male participants. Using a sample of university students in the USA (including both single and co-habiting students), she adapted the CTS questionnaire to include open-ended questions. She found that male students were more likely to disclose proportionately more violent incidents against them than women, a finding that if produced by a study using only the usual CTS tick box questionnaire, could be added to the list that support gender symmetry among young dating or cohabiting couples. Her qualitative data, however, found that 'men tend to upgrade women's violent behaviour . . . and that in contrast women may downgrade the significance of men's behaviour'. These findings lead her to question the validity of the CTS as an 'accurate measure of either the extent or the nature of violence in heterosexual relations' (Currie, 1998: 106–107).

In a study-based on women and men arrested for intimate partner violence offences in the USA, and which also used both qualitative and quantitative method-ologies, Melton and Belknap (2003: 346) found 'profound' gender differences:

> The differences between the quantitative and qualitative reports emphasize the problem with relying on officially collected 'check lists' or other 'bare-bones' measures of IPV [intimate partner violence] . . . the more detailed contextual accounts document greater gender differences, consistent with the feminist analysis, than do quantitative checklist.

This conclusion highlights the necessity of developing and utilising research methodologies which can contextualise both partners' use of physical, sexual and psychological violence (Allen and Forgey, 2007).

Consequences of and motivations for violence

Hamberger's (2005) detailed review of studies which used clinical samples to compare women's and men's use of violence supports this view. These studies found that in such samples (e.g. batterers' treatment programmes, A&E attendees, men and women arrested for domestic assault, couples attending marital counsel-ling), while 80% of the violence was bi-directional, there were profound differences between women's and men's perpetration of and experience of violence. They found that women were likely to experience greater psychological impact (including much higher rates of depression and post-traumatic stress disorder and anxiety), were more likely to be severely injured, and reported much higher levels of fear. Studies which explored motivations for using violence found that women were significantly more likely to use violence to 'protect themselves', while men report using violence significantly more than women 'to show the partner who is the boss' (Hamberger, 2005: 138). Swan et al. (2007) and Swan and Snow (2002; 2006) summarise the findings of this review of a wide range of clinical studies by suggesting that men tend to use violence 'to dominate and control their partners', while women 'tend to use violence to protect themselves or retaliate against prior violence' (Swan et al., 20007: 139). They point out, however, that there are a small number of women who use violence to dominate and control, and a small number of men who do not initiate violence, do not use it to control their partners, and suffer severe injuries.

Swan *et al.*, in a number of papers (Swan *et al.*, 2007; Swan and Snow, 2002, 2006), have explored the use of violence by women against their intimate partners. In their most recent paper (Swan *et al.*, 2007), they review what they describe as this 'small but growing research area'. Their review of this research leads them to the same conclusions as those drawn by Hamberger (2005) and outlined above. Like Hamberger, they suggest that the research concludes that women's violence usually occurs in the context of violence against them by their intimate partners, is usually motivated by self-defence and fear, and in situations of 'intimate terrorism' they are less likely to be perpetrators and more likely to be victims. They are also more likely to experience negative effects than men. They are rarely sexually abusive, are less likely to use violence for the purposes of coercive control and less likely to stalk their partners (Swan *et al.*, 2007). Like Hamberger (2005) they also suggest that interventions for men and women must take these gender differences into account.

These findings are remarkably similar to those of Dobash and Dobash (2004), in their study (which used both qualitative and quantitative methodologies) of 95 couples in which both parties used violence. They also concluded that women did not use violence in the context of control or coercion. Women's violence usually, though not always, occurred in the context of self-defence, and did not lead to as serious injury as men's violence. Men tended to report this violence as 'inconsequential', and they rarely if ever sought protection from the authorities.

In the *2000 Scottish Crime Survey* (The Scottish Executive 2000), it was reported that 19% of women and 8% of men had experienced 'threats' or 'force' from their partners or ex-partners. In a follow-up study, Gadd *et al.* (2002) were commissioned by the Scottish Executive to explore the nature of the abuse these men had experienced. Of the 90 men who had disclosed abuse 44 agreed to participate in the study. They found that relative to women victims, these men were less likely to have been repeatedly victimised or seriously injured. They found that the 'typical' female victim was more severely victimised, more fearful, more unhealthy and less financially independent than both the 'typical' male victim and other non victimised women. Interestingly, 13 of the 44 men said they had never experienced threats or force from their partners or ex-partners. The other 11 explained that they had misconstrued the focus of the original self-completion questionnaire, reporting incidents that were violent but not domestic. The only man in the sample to be subjected to a continuum of physical, emotional and sexual abuse was the only openly gay man interviewed. They concluded that rates of domestic violence against men in Scotland were much lower than the standard analyses of the *Scottish Crime Survey*, and that it is misleading to attribute 'victim status' to those men who explicitly indicated that they did not see themselves as 'victims of domestic violence'.

Separation violence

It is generally accepted that separation is the most dangerous time for abused women (Humphreys and Thiara, 2002). Sev'er (1997: 569–570), using Canadian victimisation statistics, concludes that 'separation presented a sixfold increase in risk to women in comparison to couples who continued to reside together' and that the rates of women killed by their intimate partners have been increasing in recent years. She finds an explanation for this increase in femicide rates in feminist theory, which, she maintains, is the most 'viable approach precisely because separations, especially when initiated by women, challenge the foundation of a male bastion: his power and control'.

Ellis and DeKeseredy (1997), while acknowledging that estrangement is a significant risk factor for serious violence, propose a more complex analysis to explain and help predict such lethality, pointing out that the vast majority of separated women are not killed by their ex-partners. They used Wilson and Daly's (1993) feminist concept of male proprietariness as a 'building block' for a theory which goes beyond the 'challenge theory', which they claim does not adequately explain this extreme violence and its absence in the majority of separated couples. Similarly, Brownridge *et al.* (2008: 132), whose analysis of Canadian statistics revealed that separated women reported nine times the prevalence of violence compared with married women, suggested that while patriarchal male gender identity was a significant predictor of violence against married women, it was not equally predictive of post separation physical violence. They concluded that such violence 'has many faces' and therefore requires more specific research into this aspect of intimate partner violence.

Why do men disappear in official statistics?

One of the commonest explanations for the clear disparity between the avowed gender symmetry of domestic violence and the invisibility of battered men in police and hospital statistics is by reference to the social stigma of admitting to being abused by one's female partner. As Steinmetz (1977/78: 503) notes 'the stigma ... which is embarrassing for beaten wives, is doubly so for beaten husbands'. Dobash and Dobash (1992: 76) counter this suggestion, citing Schwartz's (1987) analysis of the 1973–1982 US National Crime Survey Data, which found that 67.2% of men and 56.8% of women called the police after assault by their partners. They also cite Kincaid's (1982) study of family court cases in Ontario, which found that while there were 17 times as many female as male victims of domestic violence, only 22% of the women pressed charges in contrast to 40% of the men, and men were less likely to drop the charges.

Taft *et al.* (2001), using Australian data, state categorically that there is no 'empirical evidence that men are more likely than women to under-report to police, hospitals or to seek help'. Watson and Parsons' (2005: 77) Irish study found that men were more likely to tell someone about the abuse they were experiencing: 'about half of the women, compared to three quarters of the men had told someone within a year'. Data such as this clearly challenges the common perception that men are too ashamed to report violence by their partners.

Kimmel's (2002) conclusion, taking into account the limitations of the CTS-based studies, and including sexual assaults, homicides and post separation violence, is that rather than being a gender symmetrical expression of family conflict:

the gender ratio of male-perpetrated violence to female-perpetrated violence would be closer to 4:1. On the other hand, violence that is instrumental in the maintenance of control – the more systematic, persistent, and injurious type of violence – is overwhelmingly perpetrated by men, with rates captured best by crime victimization studies. More than 90% of this violence is perpetrated by men.

(Kimmel, 2002: 1358)

Policy implications

What may have added extra fervour to this 'most controversial' (Swan and Snow, 2006: 1027) debate is the belief that the outcome may have far reaching implications for women and men experiencing intimate partner violence. As Hamberger (2005: 142) points out, one of the reasons for this controversy is that identifying men and women as equally victimised could lead to the diversion of scarce resources from the protection of battered women. Saunders (2002: 1425) refers to a law suit filed by fathers' rights groups and some members of the National Coalition of Free Men in the USA, that funding for domestic violence programmes be stopped on the grounds of discrimination against men. According to Saunders, these groups rely on research reviews such as that by Fiebert (1998: 1) which state that there are '117 scholarly investigations, 94 empirical studies and 23 reviews and/or analyses, which demonstrate that women are as physically aggressive, or more aggressive, than men in their relationships with their spouses or male partners'. Kurtz (1993: 200) also refers to the policy implications of an uncritical acceptance of sexual symmetry in intimate partner violence, referring to the cut in funding for battered women's shelters, challenges in child custody hearings and individualist focus in counselling programmes for abused women. Currie (1998: 99) recounts the transfer of funding from women's shelters to establish shelters for battered men in New Hampshire – perhaps not coincidentally – home to the Family Research Laboratory which developed the CTS.

A gender neutral approach to arrest policies in the case of domestic violence has been found to have unexpectedly negative impacts for abused women themselves. In her 2001 qualitative study of the impact of gender neutral pro arrest policies in the USA, Miller (2001: 1339–1375) points out that despite a significant rise in the numbers of women arrested and charged for domestic violence, not one of her respondents (e.g. treatment providers, counsellors, shelter directors and workers, prosecutors, police, defence attorneys, public defenders, probations officers) believed that women's violence was increasing. The increase of female arrests was explained by changes in police policies and a fear of being named in a lawsuit for failure to arrest, as well as to 'men's greater awareness of how to use the criminal justice system to their advantage'.

The announcement in 2007 by the Irish Department of Justice, Equality and Law Reform to set up the new gender neutral COSC Office [National Office for the Prevention of Domestic, Sexual and Gender-Based Violence] has also been linked to lobbying by men's groups, who have relied on the gender symmetry arguments by Irish researchers (McKeown and Kidd, 2003). Such policy and practice outcomes continue to fuel the gender debate, but they appear to ignore the complexity of the emerging research evidence presented above.

Theories of difference and synthesis

Making distinctions

As noted earlier, theoretical approaches which seek to understand the extent, dynamics and directionality of intimate partner violence appear to be both mutually exclusive and antagonistic. The last decade has seen a number of theoretical and methodological developments which have been attempting to traverse these competing territories with theories of distinctions and syntheses. The first of these developments, and perhaps the best known to date, is that of Michael Johnson (1995; 2006; 2008). His 1995 paper addressed the twin issues of the conflicting evidence regarding prevalence and gender symmetry as presented by the family violence and feminist theorists (and discussed in detail in the previous section). Asking 'How on earth could two groups of social scientists come to such different conclusions?' he suggests that they are in fact analysing two different and mostly non overlapping phenomena. He calls these Common Couple Violence (CCV) and Patriarchal Terrorism (PT). He specifically explains that he rejects other more commonly used terms and uses this latter term because 'this pattern of violence is rooted in basically patriarchal ideas of male ownership of their female partners . . . and forces us to attend routinely to the historical and cultural roots of this form of family violence' (Johnson, 1995: 284). Yet in 2000 (Johnson and Ferraro, 2000) and later papers (Johnson and Leone, 2005; Johnson, 2006), he has adopted the gender neutral term 'Intimate Terrorism' for this form of relationship violence.

He identifies the major difference between the family violence and feminist findings as 'gender symmetry/asymmetry, per couple frequency, escalation and reciprocity' and points to the methodologies used in large-scale representative surveys (such as those of the NFV survey) as the fault-line in their very different findings. For example, he points out that in Straus and Gelles' (1990) second NFV survey, the average number of assaults reported per woman for one year was six, while in contrast, surveys using the same questionnaire but carried out with women in shelter accommodation found the average per year figure was in the 65–68 range. In order to reconcile such startling discrepancies in data between general population studies and studies of women accessing shelters, hospitals, police and other helping services, he distinguishes between Patriarchal Terrorism, (which conforms to the dynamics of power and control, severe violence which tends to escalate over time, causing serious injury requiring treatment, and often separation), and Common Couple Violence, which involves more minor violence and is less a product of patriarchy and more a product of the conflict issues suggested by Straus and his colleagues (1990).

Further distinctions

In his 2000–8 papers (Johnson and Ferraro, 2000; Johnson and Leone, 2005; Johnson, 2006, 2008), Johnson creates further distinctions between differing patterns of violence. Having abandoned PT for IT (Intimate Terrorism), he adds VR 'Violent Resistance' and MVC 'Mutual Violent Control' while CCV remains unchanged. He prefers the term VR to 'self-defence', which is perpetrated almost entirely by women, but admits that he 'presented no detailed analysis of its characteristics'. MVC, a substitute for the occasionally used term 'mutual combat', describes situations where two intimate terrorists battle for control, a situation that he concedes is rare and about which we know very little (Johnson and Ferraro, 2000: 950).

Graham-Kevan and Archer (2003) replicated and extended Johnson and Ferraro's (2000) study which sought to empirically identify the CCV and IT patterns of violence. Using an English mixed sex population sample, a shelter sample, and a CTS style questionnaire, which, they claim, obtained both self and partner report data for the first time in Britain, they measured physical aggression, controlling behaviour and emotional abuse. Their findings supported Johnson's earlier work and his distinctions regarding patterns of violence. As hypothesised, they found that IT was primarily perpetrated by males (87%), while CCV was almost sexually symmetric (45% male and 55% female). As predicted, 70% of all IT was experienced by the shelter population. Only 6% of CCV was found in the shelter sample, with 94% of the common couple violence in the community sample. Hypotheses regarding the escalation and severity in IT were also supported, as were the relationship between physical aggression and coercion. The finding that VR was almost exclusively female (90%) also supports the distinctions between male and female aggression in relationships. These findings led Graham-Kevan and Archer (2003) to conclude that patriarchal terrorism and common couple violence differ significantly in levels of physical violence, injuries, fear and controlling behaviours.

Support for these distinctions

The Bradley *et al.* (2002) Irish study would also support this contention. In this study, carried out with a sample of female patients at GP surgeries, they found that for the two-fifths of the sample who had experienced domestic violence, fear of their partner 'was significantly associated with domestic violence'. Their findings led them to conclude that asking women 'about fear and controlling behaviours' may be a more effective way of identifying women experiencing domestic abuse than simply asking about physical injuries.

The Rosen *et al.* (2005) qualitative study also examined the validity of Johnson and Ferraro's (2000) typology. They recruited a small sample of couples experiencing marital conflict through public advertisements and, despite some acknowledged difficulties, were able to categorise the couples into four separate types of intimate partner violence. The majority, 11 of the 15, were categorised as examples of CCV, one couple as MVC, two as VR. Not surprisingly, as the small sample was drawn from a community sample, and both partners had to agree to participate, they could not classify any couple as IT. They did, however, introduce a new typology, 'Pseudo-Intimate Terrorism (PIT): because one partner (the female) exercised coercive control over her male partner, she did not use 'severe violence' and he did not report great fear. This supports the studies of women's violence discussed above, in which men do not experience elevated levels of fear (Swan *et al.*, 2007; Hamberger, 2005). Given the difficulty these researchers had in identifying some of the couples in an appropriate typology, they are correct to conclude that, if these typologies are to be helpful to practitioners, they must be clear enough to be useful in making clinical and judicial decisions. Different types of violence will need different types of interventions, and no one single factor can explain all types of intimate violence (Rosen *et al.*, 2005: 330).

Johnson himself-published two studies to investigate the validity of his intimate partner violence typology (Johnson, 2006, 2008; Johnson and Leone, 2005). In his 2006 study, he has changed the title of the CCV to 'Situational Couple Violence' (SCV). He utilised a mixed sample (i.e. both an 'agency sample' and a general population sample) to investigate the difference in the levels of violence and control tactics between the four 'types' of violent couples (IT, VR, SCV and MVC) and found that violence was less frequent in men's situational couple violence, and less likely to escalate. There were more injuries in IT than in SCV. In men's intimate terrorism, women rarely respond with violence, while they are much more likely to respond with violence in men's SCV. He concludes that the data 'do not leave much doubt that intimate terrorism and situational couple violence are not the same phenomenon' (Johnson, 2006: 1010). In his paper with Leone (Johnson and Leone, 2005) they examined the differential effects of male intimate terrorism violence and situational couple violence. Using data from the US National Violence Against Women Survey which interviewed (by telephone) 8,005 men and 8,000 women, they concluded that there was a clear difference in the consequences for women from both forms of violence. Women who experience IT are attacked more frequently, the violence is less likely to stop, they are more likely to be injured and to suffer post-traumatic stress syndrome, to use painkillers and to miss work. They are also more likely to leave their partners and to find their own residences or other places of safety when they leave.

The findings of the studies reviewed in this section have implications for practice at two levels: firstly they suggest that accurate assessment of the typology of violence is essential before appropriate interventions can be made, and secondly, they suggest that mono causal explanations of violence between intimate partners are not appropriate. While it is clear from the research discussed above that coercive control and the wish to control one's partner is the primary cause of intimate partner violence, poverty and alcohol use may make this violence more severe and more life threatening. Accurate assessments and appropriate questions are essential elements in professional interventions, which can lead to effective interventions which will enhance the safety of women and children.

Women's responses to intimate partner violence

Phases of disengagement

Another area of professionals' responses to abuse is the commonly heard comment that 'women should just leave' abusive partners. To many professionals this seems to make sense, yet as was seen above, the most dangerous time for a woman is when she is about to separate. There are other reasons also why women do not leave and these will be discussed below. Liz Kelly (1988; 1994; 1995; 1996; 2005) has made a number of important contributions to contemporary understandings of intimate partner violence. Her conceptual framework of the journey women take from the time when abuse begins in their relationship to the time when violence ends is extremely helpful in trying to understand why women do not leave a relationship as soon as abuse begins. In this framework, Kelly recognises that what is done at a time of crisis can either enhance or diminish an individual's coping mechanism, and therefore must be informed by an awareness of coping strategies which they have previously or are currently employing. Kelly emphasises that whatever action is taken (which may or may not involve taking criminal or civil proceedings) it must be premised on the requirement that 'it shifts the dynamics of power and control in the woman's favour'. She outlines the variety of strategies which women use to cope with interpersonal violence, both defensive and assertive strategies and which lead her to reject the simplistic dichotomy between 'victim' and 'survivor'. She suggests that as women negotiate their responses to safety they move through a number of 'processes' (which she stresses are not 'stages', as they do not represent an orderly progression, but are more fluid) from the time the first episode of abuse occurs to the time they negotiate safety. Crisis interventions must therefore be appropriately tailored to the specific needs of the woman depending on which process she is engaged with. She identifies these six processes as follows:

1   *Managing the situation:* This occurs when the violence or abuse is first experienced in the relationship, and while some women leave at this point, the majority do not. Those who stay must develop strategies to manage the situation, which usually involves strategies to manage the environment (and her partner) in order to reduce the potential for conflict.
2   *Distortion of perspective:* As the violence continues, her daily routine becomes dominated by the need to continue to manage the situation, and will involve the acceptance of responsibility for the abuse and its consequences.
3   *Defining abuse:* After a number of assaults, the woman may come to define the abuse as violence, which implies naming her partner as an abuser and herself as an 'abused woman'. This involves placing responsibility for the abuse with her partner, and a recognition that the abuse is not just an 'aberration, but a recurring feature of the relationship'.
4   *Re-evaluating the relationship:* This recognition leads to a re-evaluation of the relationship, and the coping strategies continue in a changed context of meaning. It is now possible to contemplate the process of leaving either temporarily or permanently.

5 *Ending the relationship:* This process may require a number of attempts to leave as the barriers to doing so are complex. (As will be seen in other work, particularly in that of Kirkwood (1993) discussed below, the process of leaving is influenced by a number of abuse related, economic and interpersonal factors.)

6 *Ending the violence:* This is a recognition that ending a relationship does not necessarily imply an end to the violence, and may in fact lead to a greater risk of violence for women.

(Kelly, 1995)

While recognising that women move through these processes at differing paces, it is noteworthy that Kelly seems to imply that ending and leaving the relationship follows on from a re-evaluation of the relationship as violent.

Transtheoretical model of change

Burke *et al.* (2001) and Chang *et al.* (2006) have explored the usefulness of the 'transtheoretical model' (TM) (also known as the 'readiness to change' or the Stages of Change (SOC) model) developed by Prochaska and DiClemente (1982), to the experiences of women seeking to end abuse in their relationship. Prochaska *et al.* (1994) describe the stages of change and how a professional can work with a woman according to these stages. This model is outlined below.

Stages of change	Patient's belief	Professionals' 'nudging' strategies
Pre-contemplation	'My relationship is not a problem.'	Learn about the relationship. 'Tell me how you and your partner handle conflict in your relationship.'
Contemplation or ambivalence	'I know the violence is a problem, but I need to stay in the relationship.'	Discuss the ambivalence. 'What are the good things about your relationship?' 'What are the not-so-good things?' 'How would you change things if you could?'
Preparation	'The violence is a problem, and I'm planning some changes.'	Offer support and encouragement. Clarify plans. List community resources. Provide anticipatory guidance.

Action	'I am making changes to end the violence.'	Offer support and encouragement. List community resources. Provide anticipatory guidance. Review coping strategies.
Maintenance	'I have adapted to the changes.'	Offer support. Review need for community resources. Discuss coping strategies.
Reassessment	'I cannot maintain this change.'	Remain positive and encouraging. Discuss efforts learnt from the effort. Review Safety Plan. Remain open for future discussions.

(Adapted from 'Stages of change' for women affected by intimate partner violence (Prochaska *et al.*, 1994; Allen and Perttu, 2010))

In a qualitative study with 19 women, Khaw and Hardesty (2007) utilised the SOC model to trace women's decision making and actions in leaving violent relationships. In order to make the SOC model more relevant to the complex process of leaving, they incorporated the concept of 'turning points', which they claim has received 'scant attention' in the domestic violence literature to date (Khaw and Hardesty, 2007: 415). Using both these concepts, they identified three different trajectories of leaving abusive relationships. However, as the SOC/TM was developed for the assessment of addiction and problem drinking, the utilisation of terminology such as 'relapse' when the woman returns to the 'problem behaviour' (Khaw and Hardesty, 2007: 422) appears to reinforce a pathologising and woman blaming perspective. Chang *et al.* (2006) concluded that stage-based models may not be appropriate because of the 'non linear' process of leaving abusive partners. Anderson and Saunders (2003: 177) point out that the model is likely to be of little help to women who may wish to achieve safety and still remain in the relationship.

Leaving as process

Kirkwood (1993) utilises the 'leaving as process' approach to women's efforts to seek safety from abuse. Kirkwood's (1993) study, using data from a sample of British and US women, examines in detail the effects of emotional and physical abuse on women's journeys out of an abusive relationship and on the challenges they face in rebuilding their lives as separated/single women. Uniquely in such studies, she emphasises this latter aspect because 'the social context of abuse does not simply affect women who are being abused but also is experienced by women who have acted to free themselves from abuse' (Kirkwood, 1993: 33).

'Web'

Kirkwood (1993) proposes the analogy of a 'web', to analyse both the experience of an abusive relationship and the complex journey that women take in seeking safety and escaping the relationship (Kirkwood, 1993: 58). She utilises the analogy of inward and outward spirals within the web to describe the way in which women's strategies shift the balance of power and control between themselves and their abusers. 'Inward movement' marks an increase in control by her abuser, while 'outward movement' is marked by a decrease in control. She identifies two ways in which this change in direction can occur: firstly when the woman recognises that her self-esteem and self-worth are being damaged, or that her physical wellbeing is being threatened, and secondly, when there is a change in her energy level, which she believes can often lead to the woman leaving the relationship. This change can be motivated by anger or fear, which is accompanied by the need for self-preservation or protection for her children. Inward and outward movement along this spiral are not mutually exclusive, as a woman may be moving outward in one sphere (e.g. economic), and inward on another (e.g. diminished social contact). It is likely, as she points out, that outward movements will elicit responses from the abuser which will serve to pull the woman into an inward spiral again. She emphasises that this model of the web and the bi-directional spiralling movements are not meant to be used as 'assessment tools', or in any way to suggest that there is a normative pattern that all women must follow. She presents the model as a means of depicting the complexity and 'the depth of the process' that women in her study described.

Kirkwood's study is helpful in drawing attention to the effects of emotional abuse on women's efforts to seek safety, and to the fact that these efforts are not represented by one single decisive moment or action. Leaving abusive partners is a process rather than an event, and is influenced both before leaving and for a considerable amount of time after leaving, by the effects of the emotional and physical abuse, as well as by the influences of the social networks, both personal and public, which she reports 'were largely described as judgemental or dismissive' (Kirkwood, 1993: 132). As Anderson and Saunders (2003: 172) comment, in their review of 28 qualitative studies and 23 quantitative studies which have explored the issues that women face when leaving abusive relationships, the question that requires an explanation is 'How does she ever manage to leave given all the strikes against her?'

Nested ecological approach

In her work, 'The Battered Woman's Strategic Response to Violence' (1996) Mary Ann Dutton also examines the intricate process involved in women's decision making in response to domestic violence. She proposes a 'nested ecological approach' to clarify the multiple and intersecting influences on women's helpseeking and decision making in response to intimate partner abuse. Recognising that using a nested ecological approach is not new to the understanding of violent behaviour, Dutton insists that both individual and social factors must be taken into account when attempting to understand battered women's strategic responses to these experiences. In taking this approach, she strongly rejects the 'battered woman syndrome' concept (which grew out of Walker's (1984) 'learned helplessness' theory (discussed in Chapter 2) suggesting that such a syndrome 'gives the appearance of pathology' and ignores individual differences between women.

Dutton presents her model as an adaptation of Edelson and Tolman's (1992) model for explaining intimate violent behaviour, which includes five overlapping systems. To these five ontogenic, micro level, and macro level systems she adds an 'economic and tangible resources' variable and presents these six levels of analysis, together with relevant contextual variables, as a comprehensive model to understand individual women's responses to violence. She is clear that this model does not assume to explain a battered woman's behaviour. Rather it establishes a mechanism to understand individual differences in women's behaviour through an understanding of the factors that serve as 'either obstacles or supports in the woman's life situation' (Dutton, 1996: 118). In pointing out the implications of contextual analysis for research into women's experience, she suggests that the complexity of such an analysis may require qualitative models of research.

Women who choose to stay

The Peled *et al.* (2000) paper, in which they propose an empowerment-based ecological model of women who choose to stay in violent relationships, is an interesting counterpoint to Kirkwood's study discussed above. While Kirkwood's study emphasises the emotional and physical havoc caused by intimate partner abuse and violence and the barriers that both this abuse and wider social networks present to women leaving these relationships, Peled *et al.* theorise that the dominant professional and public discourse stigmatises battered women who stay in relationships as 'a deviant group' (Peled *et al.*, 2000: 9). Their paper (which is theoretical rather than research-based) argues that the task of giving social recognition to the problem of violence against women has led to a simplification and homogenisation of the issues involved. They point out that as 'the notion of victimization resonates with traditional gender stereotypes, it may have further fostered the image of the passive battered woman, along with the belief that overcoming such passivity necessarily involves leaving the abuser' (Peled *et al.*, 2000: 15) They recognise that the discourse of leaving is also influenced by the legal and ethical implications of, for example, social workers, who may be held liable for serious physical injuries in cases where they do not encourage women to leave.

Peled *et al.* (2000) propose that if one takes an empowerment-based approach to working with abused women, one can see the act of staying with, or returning to, an abuser as an act of choice reflecting freedom, rather than entrapment or coercion. Like Dutton (1996) discussed above, they base their ecological approach on Edelson and Tolman's (1992) model, using their four levels, (Societal-Cultural, Institutional-Organizational, Interpersonal, and Individual) as the systems within which meaning and reality are constructed, meanings which either support leaving or staying as the most appropriate options for women. However, they make a point of emphasising that these options are not static positions, but rather represent 'a tendency toward' leaving or staying (Edelson and Tolman, 1992: 19). While these 'tendencies' might be perceived by Kirkwood (1993: 78) as moving inward or outward on the spiral, with the ultimate goal of 'breaking free from abuse', Peled *et al.*, (2000) on the other hand present them as choices, which women, in the process of becoming empowered, can exercise and which may shift their partner's perception of them 'from a weak and easy prey to a strong and competent survivor whose decisions are to be respected' (Peled *et al.*, 2000: 18).

Conclusion

This chapter has explored the current debate about whether women in intimate relationships are as violent to men as some research has suggested. It should be clear from the research presented above that while a small number women are abusive, their form of abuse is different, they are not intending to control their partners (for the most part), and do not engender as many injuries or fear in their partners. Awareness of this research is important for professionals to understand, as many abusive men will blame their partners for the abuse which they themselves are inflicting on their female partners. The process of leaving is another controversial aspect of domestic violence. The five models of women's responses to leaving (or staying) in an abusive relationship, outline the complexity of this process. They add to the difficulty that many professionals experience when working with abused women, and they require a detailed understanding of the difficulty that women experience when contemplating how to deal with abuse. As was seen above, the most dangerous time for a woman is if she is contemplating separation, and she will be aware of this. As outlined in the research, each woman will react differently, and at a different pace. Social workers and other professionals working with abused women need to be aware of these complexities, and not expect all women to respond in the same way. Listening to women, hearing their understanding of their experiences, and making them aware of where they can receive specialist support is essential if abused women are not to be further controlled by those in a professional capacity.

4 Resistance responses to abuse and understanding assessment instruments

> Everyday forms of resistance make no headlines. But just as millions of anthozoan polyps create, willy-nilly, a coral reef, so do the multiple acts of peasant insubordination and evasion create political and economic barrier reefs of their own.
>
> (James C. Scott, 1985: xvii)

The previous chapters have explored many of the controversies which have made professional interventions in social work complex and difficult. This chapter will further this discussion by exploring alternative perspectives and responses to such violence by abused women themselves. It will explore the emerging literature on the increasing recognition of resistance to oppression and abuse. It will begin by presenting an overview of a range of alternative analyses of women's own responses to the experience of intimate partner violence. Anderson and Saunders (2003: 172–176) describe these qualitative approaches to women's responses and decision making in the face of abuse as 'leaving as process' studies, which focus on the woman as survivor rather than victim.

The use of the concept of 'resistance' to describe women's responses to their victimisation has been evident in the literature for almost twenty years. The first two important contributions to the discourse of women's resistance appeared in 1988. Gondolf and Fisher's *Battered Women as Survivors* (1988), a study of 6,000 women in Texas, challenged the then prevailing theory of learned helplessness, popularised by Lenora Walker's influential *The Battered Woman* (1979) and *The Battered Woman Syndrome* (1984) (discussed in Chapter 2). Gondolf and Fisher (1988: 3) concluded that 'battered women demonstrate tremendous resilience, persistence, and strengths which press for a less pathological orientation to "victims" . . . we suggest that their experience points to an alternate characterization- one that considers battered women fundamentally as "survivors"'.

Liz Kelly's *Surviving Sexual Violence*, which was also published in 1988, takes a similar approach to that of Gondolf and Fisher by drawing attention to the range of ways women resist and cope with sexual abuse and domestic violence. She defines resisting as 'to oppose actively, to fight, to refuse to co-operate with or to submit', and suggests that it involves women's refusal to be controlled (Kelly, 1988: 161). She distinguishes between coping and resistance, and between victims and survivors, suggesting that the term 'victim' makes invisible the active and positive ways in which women resist, cope and survive. Without this alternative perspective women can be presented as 'inevitably passive victims' (Kelly, 1988: 163).

Quantifying resistance strategies

In a paper published in 2003, Goodman *et al.* develop an approach to understanding and documenting women's responses to abuse, utilising a quantitative methodology to enumerate these responses. They propose what they term the 'Intimate Partner Violence Strategies Index' to investigate what factors influence women's use of defensive and resistant strategies and the effectiveness of these strategies in ensuring their safety. The index was developed as part of a longitudinal study of 406 women in the Eastern United States, and divided the helpseeking and resistance responses of abused women into six categories: placating, resistance, safety planning, legal, formal and informal. Allocating each of the responses of the women into one or other of these categories (e.g. fighting back as 'resistance', and getting help from her employer as 'formal'), unsurprisingly they found that women were more likely to use 'private strategies', which they subdivided as either placating or resistance, rather than public strategies such as seeking legal or formal help (Goodman *et al.*, 2003: 179). They found that women progressed from using private strategies to more public and formal strategies as the violence increased, but did not substitute one for the other. The strategy that was found to be most helpful by 78.9% of the respondents was that of talking to someone in a specialised domestic violence service. Goodman *et al.* (2003) found that the private forms of resistance which attempted to change the balance of power in the relationship (e.g. fighting back, or trying to end the relationship) were rated as relatively unhelpful by the women. Their overall conclusion was that public strategies which involved family, friends or formal agencies were the most helpful in terms of ending the violence. However, the use of such forms of resistance may serve functions other than simply that of ending the violence. The roles of deeper and more complex meanings and motivations need to be recognised as integral aspects of women's responses and resistances to relationship abuse.

Risk of reabuse

In a later paper based on data from the same longitudinal study, Goodman *et al.* (2005) explored the interrelationship of variables such as social support, access to individual resources and the use of resistance and placating strategies on women's safety, to their risk of reabuse. They confirmed the findings of earlier studies (e.g. Kirkwood, 1993; Goodman *et al.*, 1999; Cazenave and Straus, 1979) on the importance of the protective role of support from family and friends in reducing the risk of violence and reabuse. Similarly, they confirmed earlier studies which found that women who were employed or had their own independent homes were less likely to report reabuse. They also found that the use of placating and resistance strategies did not reduce the risk of reabuse. They found that 'women reporting high use of resistance strategies were 2.3 times more likely to be reabused'. Their explanatory hypothesis for this surprising finding is grounded in a feminist analysis of male violence, which suggests that when women attempt to challenge and subvert their partner's control, the latter will redouble their efforts to maintain that control through the use of even greater violence.

Discourses of resistance

Researchers such as Hyden (1994; 1999; 2005), Wade (1997; 2000; 2007), Coates and Wade (2004), and Todd and Wade (2003), writing from the postmodern perspective, approach the topic of resistance to violence from a less quantitative vantage point. One of the implications of postmodernism's concept of 'deconstruction of discourse' is to bring to greater awareness of the use of language in the construction of both victims and perpetrators in the context of violence and abuse. Wade (1997; 2000) and Todd and Wade (2003) draw attention to the implications of language in therapeutic interventions with victims of abuse. In his own work (1997; 2007) and in his co-authored work (Coates and Wade, 2004) Wade points out that traditional psychotherapeutic approaches tend to pathologise the abused as passive, depressed or disturbed victims, and, with few exceptions, ignore their consistent use of 'prudent, creative and determined resistance' (Wade, 1997: 23–26). He refers to Kelly's work, particularly her *Surviving Sexual Violence* (1988) as an important influence in his work on focusing on resistance in therapeutic work with victims. He rejects both the traditional Western view of resistance as typically-based on the 'male-to-male combat' – a view which excludes most forms of resistance – and the traditional psychoanalytic understanding which sees it as failure to comply with professionals' advice. His understanding of resistance is that it includes 'any attempt to imagine or establish a life-based on respect and equality'. Using accounts of his work with women who had experienced abuse, he illustrates how the choice of questions and the facilitation of in-depth discussion of reactions to this abuse enables clients to recognise their reactions and behaviours as histories of resistance to, and rejection of, the abuse they experienced. Such an approach clearly takes a broader and less rigid definition of resistance than that of Goodman *et al.* (2003) described above.

Language of resistance v. language of effects

Todd and Wade (2003) developed this approach and provide more detailed explanations of the kinds of therapeutic interventions that inform this practice. Distinguishing between the 'language of effects' and 'the language of resistance' (Todd and Wade, 2003: 159), they demonstrate how professional discourses have traditionally concealed and obscured violence and blamed or pathologised victims. Recognising the strategic need to emphasise the effects of violence on women and children as a means of counteracting social myths and conventional treatment models, they suggest that this emphasis 'encodes a number of interpretive biases ... which misrepresent victims' responses to violence' (Todd and Wade, 2003: 7).

Resistance, on the other hand, is a response that cannot be encoded in the language of effects, but it can be, and usually is, transformed into problems or symptoms or other negative end states. Using further case examples, they demonstrate how depression can be 're-heard' as a form of protest, symbolic of a refusal to be content with abuse, rather than a psychological disorder caused by the abuse. Wade (2007: 66) cites bell hooks (1990: 341) who suggests that it is necessary to locate resistance in the experience of 'despair' of marginalised people. These 'response-based' approaches are modifications of solution focused, systemic, feminist- and narrative-based approaches to therapy (Wade, 2007).

Resistance in action

John McGahern's dominant and abusive father has been referred to in Chapter 2 as an example of the expectations of 'male privilege' which is central to the feminist analysis of domestic violence (Dobash and Dobash, 1979, 1992). McGahern's mother, however, is an example of the subtle exercise of resistance to control and domination. The following short extract from McGahern's *Memoir* (2005: 92) refers to his mother's resistance to her husband's demands about her choice of a convalescence home after her treatment for cancer:

> He wanted her to go to the Boyle Nursing Home where Dympna was born because it would be less expensive than Dublin. This she refused to do. Maggie accompanied her to Dublin but she had to be careful to allay his suspicions that she was taking advice from her and others and not from him.

McGahern's (2005) *Memoir* is an enthralling account of abuse and control of both women and children by a man who expects deference and power in his relationships. Parallel to this claim to dominance is his mother's quiet but persistent refusal to be dominated. Her constant small subterfuges, as well as her occasional outright defiance, were facilitated by her economic independence as a primary school teacher. The importance of this independence is underlined by her husband's efforts to get her to resign this post when she became ill, despite his continual concerns about money. Her refusal to succumb to his demands on this issue reflects the findings of much academic work on the importance of women's economic position in their ability to resist domestic abuse (Wilcox, 2006; Kelleher and Associates, 1995). Written eloquently and dispassionately from the vantage point of a son who witnessed these patterns of behaviour, rather than from an academic or research perspective, *Memoir* (McGahern, 2005) is a powerful and classic testament to Wade's (1997; 2007) contention that resistance to abuse is ubiquitous.

Agency and positioning

Hyden (2005) introduces her paper on women's narratives of leaving with a quotation from Foucault (1980: 142) regarding the inseparability of power and resistance: 'There are no relations of power without resistance ... resistance is multiple and can be integrated in global strategies'. This quotation sets the scene for her exploration of women's narratives of leaving violent relationships in which she identifies a range of subject positions through which women recount their responses to the violence. Though she does not cite Wade, she begins her paper by stating a position very similar to his understanding of the ubiquitous nature of resistance in situations of intimate partner violence, but goes further, in that she urges feminists to include women's strategies of resistance in theorising about men's violence against women.

Hyden (2005) presents the findings of her longitudinal study (over two years) of 10 Swedish and Nordic women who were users of a centre for battered women. Her data highlights the way in which the women located themselves as actors in the process of leaving, identifying three storylines in their narratives, which correspond to three 'subject positions': 'the Wounded, the Self-Blaming and the Bridge-building' (Hyden, 2005: 176). Almost all of the women she interviewed spoke from both the Wounded and Self-Blaming positions, with some abandoning them and moving to the Bridge-building position. The characteristics of the 'Self-Blaming' position are a complex and ambiguous relationship to compliance and resistance, in which the 'woman who left' holds the 'woman who stayed' responsible for her poor judgement and responses. Only a few women spoke from the Bridge-building position, and Hyden (2005) surmises that this may be a time factor, and that more women will move to this position as time passes. In this position women are reaching out to the 'self of the past from the self of the present' (Hyden, 2005: 184) in a forgiving way, thereby building a bridge between the two subject positions. Amongst the characteristics of this position is the ambiguous nature of the woman's acts of resistance because of her inability to care for her own needs, an ability which is now increasing.

Women's helpseeking

Studies which seek to delineate the patterns of women's helpseeking generally rely on evidence from studies with women in refuge services (Binney *et al.*, 1988; Dobash and Dobash, 1985; Ruddle and O'Connor, 1992), or on analysis of social workers' caseloads (Holt, 2003). The former can be assumed to be populations experiencing severe levels of violence over a sustained period of time.

National prevalence studies: patterns of helpseeking

It will be helpful to note the patterns of helpseeking reported in both Kelleher and Associates' (1995) and Watson and Parsons' (2005) Irish prevalence studies. The sources of help and support accessed by women in these studies were strikingly similar. In both studies friends and families were reported as being the most likely to be told about the abuse: 49% and 43% respectively in Watson and Parsons (2005) and 50% and 37% respectively in Kelleher and Associates (1995). Amongst formal agencies approached, general practitioners and the Gardai were the most often sought out in both studies. Interestingly, while only 6% of women in 2005 reported the abuse to someone in the Health Board, only 7% called a helpline and 4% approached a specialist support service. Kelleher and Associates reported that in their national survey, only 2% approached a social worker for help. Their findings in the area-based study carried out with women in doctors' surgeries (as part of the national study) found a considerable difference in the figures regarding social work contact. Of the 56 women who had reported their experience of violence 24 did so to the social services, ahead of doctors, the court system, priests/ministers or refuges. This reflects the findings of Dobash and Dobash (1985) and Bowker (1983) which show that contact with social services is likely to increase as the level of violence (and therefore injury) increases.

Women's resistant responses to abuse

In a study carried out by Allen (2012b) the narratives of the participants provide enormously rich data which elucidates the range of strategies in which the women engaged as responses to their partners' abusive behaviours. The data clearly supports Coates and Wade's (2004) contention that 'resistance to violence is ubiquitous' and also demonstrates the accuracy of the Goodman *et al.* (2003) comprehensive list of resistant strategies. The following extracts provide some examples of this 'ubiquitous' resistance by the study participants.

All of the women in Allen's study engaged in a number of highly sophisticated strategies either to avoid an outburst or an escalation of the situation, or to minimise the effect of the abusive behaviour on themselves or their children. Because the data contains so many examples of resistant responses, they have been subdivided into a number of subcategories which illustrate the range of strategies involved. They are presented in ascending order of 'confrontational' intent. By confrontational intent is meant the extent to which the behaviour can be seen as a direct challenge to her partner's actions, and usually progresses from avoidance, through verbal disagreement or challenge to outright physical retaliation.

Avoidance

Frances: I just ignored it, that kind of way. You know, I'd deal with it there and then, and two minutes afterwards, when it was all over, it went to the back of my head.

Rose: Now I'd know better than to open my mouth to him.

Susan: And I stopped watching my favourite programmes, but because he was getting so annoyed.

Managing him

Rose: So the more he treated me like that, the better I tried to treat him, so that he would treat me the way I wanted to be treated.

Frances: He'd say either do it my way, or don't do it at all. That's when I decided
to let him take over the relationship, so to speak, to keep him happy.

These extracts suggest that Frances and Rose (and all the other women in the study)
are strategically changing their behaviour to avoid abuse, or even more strategically,
to change their partners' patterns of behaviour. Campbell *et al.* (1998: 755) describe
this strategy of resistance as 'subordinating the self', which they classify as both a
proactive, conscious choice and a defensive strategy to avoid further abuse, as
described above by Frances and Rose. Taken in isolation, however, Frances's
comment could be understood as passivity or even 'helplessness', but her responses,
far from exhibiting helplessness, demonstrate a 'strongwilled' and 'stubborn'
woman who engaged in a variety of resistant responses in an increasingly abusive
relationship, resulting finally in legal action, separation and safety.

Verbal confrontation

The most frequently cited form of resistance in these narratives can be described
as 'verbal confrontation'. This form of response encompasses a variety of verbal
tactics to resist and challenge what the women experienced as unreasonable, irra-
tional or threatening behaviour. A small sample of such responses is illustrative of
some of these strategies:

Margaret: I was trying to stand to argue my point with him . . .
Phil: He came in and said something about his dinner, and I said 'dinner,
with what? There's no money'. I'd paid for the ESB [Electricity
Supply Board] and shoes or whatever was needed, and there was no
money for dinner left. And he said, 'I'll have me dinner'. I said, you
go and buy it and cook it.
Susan: And I said, you're not working, you haven't got the money. If you'd
let me work, we might have a little bit more money and it'd make
things a little bit more easy.

Strike action

Downing tools and refusing to cooperate with the demands of their partner was
another form of resistance utilised by the participants.

Phil: . . . normal day-to-day cleaning I'd do, but not a [drinking] session like
that – I'd say to him, if you've a session, you clean it up.
Ann: I went on strike that particular day . . . I think something snapped, and he
wanted the place shipshape, and I said no, I'm not doing it. Not any more.
So they all helped to tidy up – and I thought this was great. When I looked
back on it I thought, God, they're actually doing something. And I sat
there and I read a book or something.

Subterfuge

Subterfuge is a response which straddles the categories of 'resistance and agency'. Once again there are a number of examples of this form of response by the women, in which they take independent action without their partners' knowledge or consent. In the light of the level of control and violence these women experienced, such action is often high risk behaviour and demonstrates the lack of 'helplessness' in their responses. What is of note in these narratives is that the most complicated subterfuge concerns issues of fertility and the control of reproduction. In view of violent men's attempts to control this aspect of their partners' lives (Campbell *et al.*, 1998) resistance to this control is of great significance. The following extract from Frances not only confirms her ability to engage in elaborate resistance, but these actions also confirm her self-identity as 'strongwilled' and 'stubborn'.

Frances: He went mad, he wanted more kids. So for about six months he was going mad over wanting another one . . . But I said no. I wasn't able for it . . . And I said to him, I had to go to the doctor and see what they could do. And I went in, and I didn't go to the doctor, but I went around the town and came out, and I said, the doctor said if I want to have it [a contraceptive device] out, I have to wait three months on the waiting list and then it could be three months after they take it out and then it could take six months before I could become pregnant. And that's what he believed then.

Frances's subterfuge demonstrates the creative use of the well-known shortcomings of the public health system! Phil faced a similar dilemma in resisting her partner's demands for another child, but in her case she actively enlisted the help of her GP in the subterfuge, who, when her partner asked him if there was 'nothing [he] could do . . . to fix her up', replied, 'I can do no more. That's it. I've sent her to Holles St. [maternity hospital] – it's in God's hands'. Not surprisingly, Phil describes her GP as 'great fun'.

Physical resistance

The use of violence by women in intimate relationships has been the source of a great deal of contemporary debate and has been discussed in some detail in Chapter 3. Much of this debate has centred on the use of violence as self-defence by abused women (Hamberger, 2005; Saunders, 2002; Swan *et al.*, 2007).

This research clearly supports the view that physical violence is one of the many forms of resistance which women call upon in their efforts to keep themselves and their children safe (Campbell *et al.*, 1998; Goodman *et al.*, 2003; Saunders, 2002). However, it appears to support only partially the findings of Goodman *et al.* (2005) that women's violence or violent resistance may contribute to an escalation of men's violence. The latter suggest that 'resistance appears to be a strong risk factor for reabuse even after taking into account severity of violence'

(Goodman *et al.*, 2005: 330). Only in the case of Rose (and to a lesser extent Frances) is it unequivocal that her use of physical confrontation resulted in an escalation of abuse:

Rose: And then the time I retaliated . . . I don't know what started it . . . and that started him off. So he took me by the hair and he threw me up against the kitchen units and he was screaming at me.

The following extracts from Margaret, demonstrate the dangers of treating the use of violence out of the context of the violent relationship:

Margaret: I gave him a black eye once, and that was purely by accident, it really was. We were fighting and he was – all this shite coming out of his mouth, crap – screaming at me. And I just went like that – across his face – and it was my ring, my engagement ring caught him in his eye, here. And he nearly went ballistic when he saw it. And I just said, now you know what it feels like to have a black eye.

Taken out of context, not just of this individual incident, but of the longstanding coercive and verbally and physically abusive nature of this relationship, this resistant action might appear as 'bi-directional violence' (Forgey and Badger, 2006) or 'situation or common couple violence' (Johnson, 2008) and illustrates the concerns (discussed in Chapter 3) regarding findings from studies using the Conflict Tactics Scale (Dobash and Dobash, 2004). Campbell *et al.* (1998: 754) found that half of the women in their study reported hitting their partner when 'fighting back'. Adding to the complexity of abused women's use of violence, it would appear Margaret's physical resistance was not limited to accidental retaliation. In this extract she uses 'strategic' injury, and, as in the former extract, accompanies the physical response with verbal resistance:

Margaret: I actually kicked him in the 'altogether' to get him off me, because he was on top of me on the bed. And he screamed at me, don't you ever do that to me again. He says, look at what you keep making me do! And I said, . . . I never asked you to punch the head off me. I'm not asking you to do any of that, you're doing it.

The narratives show that all of the women (with the exception of Ann who experienced the least physical abuse) engaged in physical resistance to abuse. Lorraine, who experienced extreme physical abuse, contemplated the ultimate form of physical resistance – murdering her partner while he was asleep.

Lorraine: I was sitting on the other bed, like this, with a hammer. And he was asleep like that, so I was thinking of getting him – and I was sitting there and I would stand up, and I'd say, no, what if he'd wake up . . . and then over in England . . . I was planning on stabbing him . . .

This level of resistance, even though it was not actually carried through, demonstrates the extent of resistant responses which abused women will at least contemplate in their efforts to keep themselves safe from further violence. It also demonstrates her sense of self-preservation in her awareness of the consequences if she did not 'complete' the job.

The strategy of leaving

All of the participants in this study were forced to leave their homes on one or more occasions as a result of their abusive experiences. Some, like Ann and Liz, left a number of times, usually staying with friends, and finally, staying in a women's refuge until they secured permanent rehousing on their own. Others, for example Susan, made one final break, also staying in a refuge for a short period of time.

Susan: I'm afraid to be in the house on my own. So, anyway, I went in there [refuge], went home and packed up stuff – terrified that he's going to find me.

Brenda: When I was after getting the Protection Order, and they [police] told me to stay out of the house. I wasn't to go back . . . Their advice was, he's after flipping now he knows you have the Protection Order.

The strategy of leaving an abusive partner has been described by Kirkwood (1993: 66) as the 'outward movement on the web' taking the woman away from the centre where her partner exerts total power and control. It can be described as the ultimate form of resistance, but as Campbell *et al.* (1998), and the narratives of Brenda and Frances in particular, make clear, it is not synonymous with ensuring safety from violence. The pervasive nature of post separation violence has been one of the arguments discussed in Chapter 3 to identify the particular dynamics of male to female intimate violence and it describes leaving as a strategy which challenges the 'gendered' stereotypes of victimhood, referring particularly to women who return and remain in the relationship. It is impossible to be exact about the proportion of abused women who leave violent relationships, as the assessment of such responses depends entirely on the moment in time when one asks each particular woman about this option. However, the findings of the anonymous national prevalence Watson and Parsons (2005: 70) study support the suggestion that the majority of abused women do eventually end an abusive relationship, but this may be preceded by women leaving and returning more than once (Anderson and Saunders, 2003; Peled *et al.*, 2000). As the analysis of this study makes clear, the resistant responses of these women occurred throughout the lifetime of the abusive relationship, and leaving (even temporarily) is but one amongst many resistance strategies. As Anderson and Saunders (2003: 176) suggest, temporary separations give women the autonomy and self-confidence to make a 'final break'.

It is, however, almost the accepted wisdom of professionals who encounter women experiencing abuse, to assume that leaving is the best option for an abused woman, and their interventions are usually focused on her doing so as quickly as possible. Notwithstanding the wisdom of such interventions in times of great danger, the resistance of women to this form of directive intervention is often a source of bewilderment, if not outright annoyance, on the part of social workers and other professionals and family members who wish to ensure her safety. However, the strategies of resistance which abused women use need to be understood in order to fully understand the complex nature of her responses, her wishes for the relationship and her level of fear if she does leave.

Assessment tools

In order to make sense of women's use of resistance, their level of fear and their wishes for their relationship, it is important that social workers make accurate assessments of the experiences of abused women and children. However, there is no one assessment 'instrument' that is universally accepted by all social workers. Some agencies use such instruments, and others feel that they are not necessary. The following sections will outline a number of such instruments, some of which are free to the user, but many others (not listed here) which have to be paid for. As Humphreys and Stanley (2006) point out, various studies have shown that women are unlikely to disclose domestic violence unless they can be assured that the reaction will be positive – that is not woman blaming or taking children into care.

Using assessment and screening tools

The issues one needs to establish when making assessments of the level of danger a woman may be facing involve the following elements:

- frequency/level of violence/over what time period;
- types of violence – psychological, physical, sexual;
- consequences of violence – fear/anxiety/injuries, etc.;
- what happens between violent episodes – control, decision making, isolation, etc. (Power and Control Wheel, see Figure 1.1);
- substance abuse/dependency;
- her resistance strategies;
- involvement of children – direct/indirect targets (be aware this will cause anxiety).

Enabling clients to disclose abuse may be difficult. Initially it may be helpful to approach the client by asking non-threatening questions in an empathetic manner. For example:

- 'Is everything all right at home?'
- 'How are you feeling?'
- 'Are you getting the support you need at home?'

- 'I noticed X, Y and Z and I am concerned about you. I wonder if there is anything I can do to help?'
- 'You seem afraid. Is there something you would like to talk about?'

If the client affirms that there are problems at home, is hesitant or gives an answer which causes concern, social workers (and nursing or other professionals) should *always* investigate further.

Screening questionnaire

Most women do not disclose being victims of intimate partner violence to health or social work professionals even though they most often seek help from them. Since the majority of health professionals do not ask about intimate partner violence most cases remain unnoticed. Screening questionnaires-based on the experience of health professionals are helpful in asking about violence in intimate relationships and about violence against children. The screening questionnaire, of which excerpts are included below, is based on Finnish research and the Abuse Assessment Screen (AAS) (McFarlane and Parker, 1994). This screening questionnaire focuses on the behaviour of the current partner. In addition to physical and sexual violence, questions about controlling behaviour and psychological violence are included, since those often lead to physical violence and/or there are signs of physical and/or sexual violence.

The screening questionnaire also contains questions about the children's experience as witnesses of partnership violence (seeing or hearing) and violence against the children themselves. The need for further help is also checked in the questionnaire in order to be able to continue the support.

Examples of direct questions

- 'Are you or have you ever been afraid of your partner?'
- 'You seem frightened of your partner, has your partner ever hurt you?'
- 'Do you feel, or have you felt unsafe at home?'
- 'Is there someone making you afraid?'
- 'Does your partner try to control you?'
- 'Have you been hurt or threatened by your partner or a family member?'
- 'Is there anybody you know that caused you injury?'
- 'How have they hurt you?'
- 'Have they hurt you physically, sexually, emotionally?'
- 'When did they hurt you?'
- 'You mention that your partner loses his temper with the children, does he lose his temper with you?'
- 'Many women who come to us experience some form of emotional or physical abuse at home. Has this happened to you?'

Gently challenge the woman if the injuries do not fit with the explanation given:

- 'I notice you have a number of bruises, could you tell me how that happened, did someone hit you?'
- 'When I see these marks, they are more usually the result of being struck. Has anyone hit you?'

Adapted from Allen and Perttu (2010)

The Mental Health Services in the West of Ireland use a short screening questionnaire to establish if women are being abused (abuse can lead to high levels of depression and suicide attempts). This questionnaire (Figure 4.1) builds up from

---

Suggested questions for asking about domestic violence

These questions can be used at an initial meeting with a client or at a later time:

1. What happens when you have an argument or row at home? Does anyone criticise you, make fun of you or call you names?

2. Do you ever feel unsafe in your own home? Have the Gardai ever been called to your home due to a domestic disturbance?

3. Are you ever prevented from leaving your home, seeing your friends or family; prohibited from getting a job, socialising, or owning your own money?

4. Is there someone at home jealous or possessive of you, for example questioning your movements, checking your whereabouts, following you, believing you have other partners, checking your mobile phone, your email, computer use history or post?

5. Have you ever had your home/possessions damaged or a family pet harmed?

6. Have you ever been threatened with a weapon, hit, kicked, or hurt in any way at home?

7. Have you ever been threatened that your children will be taken away from you?

8. Have your children overheard, witnessed or experienced domestic violence?

9. Have you ever been forced to engage in sexual acts against your will?

10. Do you feel safe going home and if not what would you need to happen to make it safe for you to do so?

11. Is there anything else that you would like to mention or add?

For practitioner use only

If there is a disclosure of domestic violence it is important to assess whether the abuse took place over a period of time, so please evaluate for a history of :

Childhood abuse ☐
Past domestic abuse ☐

Please remember to explain these points to the client:
* *Routine nature of assessment/enquiry*
* *Confidentiality policy of service*
* *Client's and their children's safety is the priority*

Is intervention necessary?   Is it immediate?   Is the referral to an outside agency?

Figure 4.1 Suggested questions for asking about domestic violence.

Source: Adapted from *HSE Mid-West Area Adult Mental Health Services Domestic Violence Assessment Tool*, 2005

disagreements to control and coercion and then to physical violence. It will require follow-up intervention if the woman discloses abuse.

These responses need to be recorded and follow-up services involved to ensure the safety of the woman and her children.

Multi Level Assessment Worksheet

Another example of domestic violence assessment is the Multi Level Assessment Worksheet.

This approach takes both the risks and the strengths of the woman into consideration and explores the individual, family and environmental risk factors and strengths. This is an approach which incorporates women's resistance and the wider cultural beliefs of the community in which the couple live. The issues to be explored include the following:

Pattern of Violence: Form(s), level, frequency, direction, motive, meaning, consequences

Individual Risk Factors	**Individual Strengths**
Family Risk Factors	**Family Strengths**
Environmental Risk Factors	**Environmental Strengths**

This approach to assessment incorporates a range of levels, as well as risks and strengths.

Suffolk Tools for Practitioners

In Suffolk in Britain, a project was initiated called the Suffolk Tools for Practitioners (Suffolk TfP; Hester and Westmarland, 2005). This project involved the training of social care workers and health visitors in using the Duluth Power and Control Wheel (outlined and discussed in Chapter 1) as a means for assessing for domestic violence. The use of the Power and Control Wheel is a very effective means of enabling a woman to identify the forms of abuse she is experiencing. This is an alternative to just being asked about physical or verbal abuse. The Power and Control Wheel enables abused women to identify forms of abuse they may not have seen as abusive or controlling. The feedback from those trained was extremely positive and adds to the evidence that both training and assessment tools can assist practitioners to enable women to disclose abuse.

Co-ordinated Action Against Domestic Abuse (CAADA)

An assessment tool that is now being used widely in Britain is that developed by CAADA (2010) as a risk identification checklist. This is quite a long questionnaire and should be used in situations where a high risk is suspected. It can be downloaded from the following website: http://www.caada.org.uk/marac/ TOOLKIT%20FIPs%20updated%20July%202010.pdf.

This checklist has 24 questions and explores the level of violence, the extent of the fear the woman is experiencing, levels of isolation from family and friends, and whether the woman is experiencing suicidal thoughts or suffering from depression. It also explores levels of jealousy, substance abuse, suicide threats by the abuser, and whether there have been abuse to a family pet, or threats to kill her or harm the children. This is a very detailed assessment tool and should be used when a woman discloses a serious level of abuse, including suicide threats or harm to children.

Instructions for the use of the screening questionnaire

- Pose the questions calmly and without hurry. Give the woman time to think about them and the possibility to ask further questions.
- You can go through the set of questions while talking. Yet, it is important that the same questions are asked in the same way. In order to do so the questions must be put (read) as they are on the form.
- Give practical examples by explaining what for example 'controlling behaviour' means.
- Specify the questions if needed.
- Document the victim's story by using her words and expressions.
- Documentation is important for her legal rights and her protection – she might need the documentation later if she wants to report to the police/go to court.
- The way you ask and write down the story is important.
- The woman has the right to read the form and to have a copy of it.

Adapted from Perttu and Kaselitz (2006)

The RAVE Study

Recognising that there is an increasing demand for accurate risk assessment in the field of domestic violence, Roehl *et al.* (2005) (in the USA) carried out a comparison of four such tools. These were: The Danger Assessment, DV-Mosaic, Domestic Violence Screening Instrument (DVSI), and the Kingston Screening Instrument for Domestic Violence (K-SID). These four methods vary in length and complexity. The purpose of the study was to assess their accuracy in predicting further violence. The participants in the study involved a range of ethnic backgrounds, levels of education, employment status and situations of whether the abuser was, or was not, cohabiting with the victim. All of the participants were women seeking help for violence from their intimate partner. They found that women participating in the study took significant steps to protect themselves from further abuse after the first interview. This is an important finding as the use of the questionnaire enabled women to see the danger they were in. Yet despite these protective actions, 31% of the women were physically abused between the baseline interviews and the follow-up interviews. Of these 56% were severely abused and seriously hurt, and 36%

experienced potentially lethal abuse. All four of the assessment tools were found to be significantly related to subsequent severity of abuse. They found that brevity and length did not correspond with accuracy. The Danger Assessment Tool performed better than the other methods, as it produced the best overall predictive model. However, they felt that without further research, practitioners need to take the following steps when working with abused women:

1   Carefully ask the victim her perception of her risk and take heed of her judgement.
2   Continue to assess risk with all means available, including the expert judgement and clinical wisdom of practitioners, including their knowledge and the offenders criminal record, a formal method with some evidence of predictive accuracy like those tested in this study, and the victim's own assessment.
3   Where victim safety is your greatest concern, use lower risk categories on formal methods to identify cases for investigation. Where offender fairness and/or scarce resources are your greatest concern, use higher risk categories to identify cases for sanctioning or intensive services.
4   Be vigilant about potential harm to victims and perpetrators, as the science of risk assessment is young.

These suggestions for making assessments should assist practitioners to take heed of women's own judgements, making sure that appropriate levels of care and intervention are instigated, and that the woman is informed of appropriate services and refuges.

Conclusion

This chapter has explored the issues of women's resistance to domestic violence and the strategies that they undertake to keep themselves safe. Examples from abused women's experiences were cited as examples of how women manage situations to keep themselves safe. Unfortunately these resistance tactics are often seen by others as simply 'giving in', but if women are listened to, and their experiences understood as resistance, social workers and other professionals are more likely to understand the actions women take to protect themselves and their children. However, the use of risk assessment tools can be extremely helpful not only in enabling a social worker to make an assessment of risk, it can also help the abused woman to recognise the level of risk she faces. Informing women of the outcome of these assessments is important for her safety and future wellbeing. There is a range of such assessments, as was seen above, some quite long, and some much shorter. However, it is important to make sure that risk assessments such as the CAADA Risk Assessment Tools or the Danger Assessment Tools are used when a woman discloses serious abuse from her partner. To ignore such assessment tools will put not only women, but their children, at increased risk of abuse and possible lethal harm.

5 Emergency and longer-term interventions

Supporting abused women requires both short-term and long-term interventions. Some abused women will come to the attention of social workers when they are in a state of crisis, others will emerge as a result of screening in a medical setting (see the following chapter), or as a result of a child protection issues (see Chapter 8). The social worker, in whichever setting s/he is located, will need to be aware of the dynamics of the abusive relationship, the immediate steps to take and the longer-term support the woman needs to ensure her safety. This chapter will explore these approaches, providing practitioners with a range of options, depending on what the woman herself feels she needs at that particular time.

Background to the development of services for abused women

The feminist analysis of intimate partner violence developed in the early 1970s (Stark, 2007: 22–23) from both feminist theorising about the role of women in society and from the 'battered women's' movements, particularly those in the USA and in Britain. The 'battered women's' movements were in turn shaped and influenced by the resulting feminist analysis. Dobash and Dobash (1992) trace the development of this movement from within feminism while acknowledging its resulting complex inter-relationship. Schechter (1982: 29) argues that it was 'no mere accident' that a ground-swell of calls to lawyers and therapists from battered women began to be heard in the 1970s, and she challenges the suggestion that 'society' had suddenly recognised this problem (Schechter, 1982: 3). She cogently argues that it was 'the emerging feminist movement' and grassroots activists who painstakingly 'detailed the conditions of daily life that would allow women to call themselves battered' (Schechter, 1982: 29).

Stark (2007: 28), cites the Women's Advocates Shelter in St. Paul, Minnesota in 1974, and Dobash and Dobash (1992: 25) cite the Chiswick refuge in London in 1971, as examples of how emergency housing projects for battered women arose from women coming together in consciousness raising groups. The first shelter in Boston, Transition House, was another example of how the emerging women's movement influenced the refuge movement. Although the two women who started the shelter were former battered women, they were soon joined by two members of Boston's earliest radical feminist groups. Abused women using the house were encouraged to explore their personal lives, learning the political parameters of 'private' problems. For the activists 'battering was an integral part of women's oppression; women's liberation its solution' (Schechter, 1982: 34).

Dobash and Dobash (1992: 25) also trace the origins of the battered women's movement directly to the wider feminist movement and contend that 'most of the early shelter groups arose out of women's liberation consciousness raising groups'. They place these developments within the radical feminist tradition of feminist thought suggesting that the 'pro-woman' orientation of that tradition 'has led to a concentration on the central importance of gender, the intimate domination of women under patriarchy and a consideration of its institutional and ideological forms' (Dobash and Dobash, 1992: 75). McLaughlin (2003) also locates concerns with women's lives in the 'private sphere' such as sexuality, reproduction, domestic labour and domestic violence in what is called the 'second wave' of feminist activism. (The second wave of feminism is generally thought to span the period from early to late twentieth-century.) 'Second wave feminism, in different ways, connected the continued gaps in the rights and opportunities women suffered in the public realm to the roles they played in the private spheres' (McLaughlin, 2003: 1).

Interventions for abused women

Women have a variety of reasons for not disclosing intimate partner violence in their relationships. Leaving a partner is the most dangerous time for a woman, and this important point needs to be kept constantly in mind by all professionals working with abused women. The reasons for not disclosing intimate partner violence can involve any of the following issues:

- fear of increased violence;
- wanting to keep the family together;
- guilt, shame, isolation, exhaustion, unpredictability;
- not wanting 'to fail' in their relationship (reinforced by family, colleagues, etc.);
- fearful because of constant threats, stalking, access arrangements, etc.;
- poor self-esteem;
- contradictory feelings;
- concern for her own safety;
- concern for her children's well being;
- belief partner can change;
- isolation and lack of resources;
- lack of assistance or services;
- financial concerns;
- economic dependence – nowhere else to go;
- structural barriers in courts, social services;
- gender roles and lack of family support;
- attitudes of the professionals;
- attitudes in the society.

(Allen and Perttu, 2010)

All of these issues need to be explored with the woman when it is appropriate to do so.

In order to ensure that a woman feels safe and can disclose the abuse to a professional who can help her the following guidelines can be helpful.

Good practice responses common to all professionals

Do

- DO provide a safe environment conducive to disclosure. (Remember if the person is accompanied by their partner it will not be safe for them to disclose.)
- DO give priority to the patient's immediate safety whether or not they leave.
- DO reassure the patient that the abuse is not their fault.
- DO let the patient know that they are not alone in being abused.
- DO refer the patient to specialist agencies and individuals.
- DO remember that the patient's options may be limited by lack of or access to resources.
- DO remember that confidentiality is crucial.
- DO check if it is safe to send her letters or to phone her at home.
- DO keep appropriate records.
- DO recognise the different needs of women with a disability or sensory impairment and have support appropriate to their specific needs.

Don't

- DON'T ignore your intuition if you suspect a woman has been abused.
- DON'T insist on joint sessions with her and the man.
- DON'T ask her if she did something to provoke the violence, just the facts. This places the responsibility of the abuse with the victim instead of the abuser.
- DON'T make decisions for her.
- DON'T expect her to leave her home or her partner.
- DON'T expect her to make life changing decisions in a hurry.
- DON'T give up on her because things are taking longer than you think they should. Dealing with intimate partner violence is a process of different stages and attempts. The relationship is not static, which means that the woman's attitude to herself, the abuse and the abuser will change over time.
- DON'T put pressure on her to disclose. It is always her choice.
- DON'T pass on information about her whereabouts to anyone without her explicit consent.

The following guidelines are specifically set out for social workers.

Good practice responses for social workers

- Take her seriously, believe her and create the necessary conditions to disclose.
- Assess immediate risk to women (and her children, if any).
- How can you facilitate this woman to ensure her safety?
- Does she require immediate access to a refuge?
- What supports are available to her at present?
- What options has she tried already?
- Make her aware of the options available – legal, financial, support services such as Women's Aid, housing, refuge, local support group, etc.
- Help her to devise an immediate and long-term safety plan.
- Link her into community and support services.
- Follow-up contact with the woman should be initiated in ways that maximise her safety. Check if it is safe to send her letters or to phone her at home.
- Recognise the different needs of women with a disability or sensory impairment or from a different cultural background and have support appropriate to their specific needs.
- Keep appropriate records.
- If children are concerned, assess the level of risk and refer to appropriate agencies.

Adapted from *Domestic Violence: A Health Issue: Guidelines for Hospital Staff*, 2004

In order to be able to provide immediate addresses and telephone numbers to a woman it is important that the social worker has these to hand. However, it is very important to remind women that leaving such information around the house where her abusive husband or partner may find it is very dangerous and may provoke even greater abuse or violence. For social workers in all settings the following outline can be completed so that urgent information can be given to women.

Local Helpline (e.g. Women's Aid)	Phone number.
Local Support Services:	Phone number and address.
Local Refuge:	Phone number and address.
Refuge in another area:	Phone number and address.
Local Police Number:	Phone number.
Local Legal Aid: (if available)	Phone number and address.
Hospitals the woman may have attended:	Phone number(s).

Legal situation

Intimate partner violence is a violation of one's human rights. Furthermore, in all EU countries it is also a crime to assault or abuse one's intimate partners. However, the legislation regarding this crime varies from country to country. As it is important for professionals to know the legal situation in their own country, they need to be given an overview of the legislation and the rights of intimate partners under the legislation. As there is a difference between the civil and criminal legislation which impacts on the legal and police action which can be taken, and the particular court system and sanctions open to abused partners, these aspects of the legislation should be outlined to students. The following are the topics with which they should be familiar:

- The Domestic Violence Legislation in their State
- Is there both Civil and Criminal Legislation: Are there Protection Orders? (i.e. Barring Orders/Exclusion Orders?)
- How can an abused partner access these Orders?
- Do they need legal representation?
- Is there free legal aid available to them?
- How can they access this Legal Aid?
- Who can the professional contact to update themselves regarding this legislation?

(Allen and Perttu, 2010)

Safety planning

It is essential to make a safety plan with all women presenting with intimate partner violence related injuries or distress, and with those who disclose such abuse. This should always be done in a collaborative, non directive manner. After having evaluated her situation and having estimated the dangerousness of the perpetrator it is important to draw up an individual safety plan together with the woman.

Discuss with the woman how she can protect herself and her children:

- Anticipating violence: Are there signs that indicate the possibility that the partner will become violent?
- Escape routes: How and where to escape/go to be safe? Which is the safest room? Where is there no exit?
- Dangerous places: The kitchen is an especially dangerous place because there are knives, etc. It is advisable to avoid bathrooms and other rooms without exit.
- Leaving the house: How to leave the house in a natural way? Empty the garbage bins, take the dog out, etc.
- Protecting oneself during a violent incident: How can she protect herself and her children? The woman can learn how to protect herself from attacks. It does not prevent violence but can reduce the seriousness of injuries.
- She should talk to the children about situations in which it might become necessary to leave home as quickly as possible. It is good to

talk about what to do in violent situations and where to escape to. She can also teach children to call emergency numbers (it would be good if they memorised these numbers). If the children are very young, the mother should find somebody to whom she could take them.

- Agreements with trustworthy neighbours/friends/relatives: Is there a neighbour to which she can escape or with whom she can hide? She can also arrange with the neighbours that they will call the police when they hear sounds of violence. Neighbours can keep the safety bag, etc.
- Advise her to make a second plan in case the first plan does not work.

Adapted from Perttu and Kaselitz, 2006

Safety plan steps

Step 1

Think about:

- Who can I call in a crisis?
- Where you can go to make a telephone call?
- A safe place where you can go to stay in an emergency. This may be a friend or relative, a women's refuge, a hotel or a B&B.
- The telephone number of a safe place.
- What are the escape routes from my house/trailer/flat?
- How to get to the safe place. Decide how you will get there at different times of day or night.
- The number of a local taxi firm.
- What to tell the children and how to tell it to them, when you need to put the safety plan into action.
- Can I work out a signal with the children and/or neighbours to call Gardaí/Police or get help? (It is important to teach the children how to call emergency services.)

Step 2

Write down (but be sure they cannot be found by your abusive partner):

- Important phone numbers:
  - taxi
  - doctor
  - police station
  - solicitor
  - district court
  - health centre (Community Welfare Officer)

- ○   social welfare office
- ○   housing department
- ○   women's refuge number
- ○   family
- ○   friends

- Your family's essential medicines
- Your PRSI/PPSN [Pay Related Social Insurance/Personal Public Service Number]
- Your child benefit book number.

Step 3

Collect together the following items. Hide them somewhere you can get them in a hurry. It may be a good idea to put them in a bag and store it with a friend.

- essential medicines;
- enough money (especially to get to a safe place by bus or taxi);
- an extra set of keys for your home, car or office;
- driving licence;
- extra clothes for you and your children (school uniforms);
- children's favourite toys/blanket;
- address and phone book.

The Health Services and Social Welfare Services require personal identification and evidence to assess your entitlement, for example:

- identification for self, e.g. birth certificate;
- children's birth certificates;
- medical card;
- PRSI/PPSN card;
- marriage certificate;
- bank book and details;
- pay slips;
- lease/rental agreement/mortgage agreement;
- passport;
- any court order or documents.

Step 4

If you can, discuss your safety plan with a trusted friend so that they can support you if you need to put it into action. Keep your safety plan in a safe place – ideally somewhere you can get it quickly and if you need to leave in a hurry.

Adapted from *Domestic Violence: A Health Issue:*
Guidelines for Hospital Staff, 2004

It is important that these safety plans are carefully worked out with the woman, keeping in mind that if found by her partner it may trigger greater violence and even homicide.

Counselling abused women

Utilising the Good Practice Guidelines, taking an accurate history of the abuse, making a risk assessment and accurately recording a woman's abuse, developing a safety plan and making the appropriate referrals are the first important steps in providing support in a clinical setting. However, in some settings, in particular in some social work settings, it may be possible to provide ongoing counselling support for an abused woman. This can also be provided in women's refuges and specialised support services for abused women (e.g. Women's Aid). A number of counselling and therapy approaches have been developed for women who experience intimate partner violence (Wade, 1997, 2007; Wood and Roche, 2001; Roche and Wood, 2005) but whichever approach is used, counselling must pay special attention to a woman's safety. Referring a couple to marriage or joint couple counselling can be dangerous and will be ineffective.

Individual counselling therefore is essential for effective and safe practice. The basic principles of a strengths perspective are appropriate when engaging in such counselling as they respect and reinforce women's own coping strategies, thereby increasing her self-esteem and self-confidence, which will enable her to make long-term decisions to ensure her own and her children's safety. Counselling, however, should not be terminated once the woman has obtained a protection order or left her partner. This is the most dangerous time for an abused woman and it is the time she will need most support. She may be intimidated by her abusive partner into returning to him, to give the relationship 'another go' or she may be harassed or stalked by him. There may be ongoing legal difficulties about access to their children. All of these issues may undermine her decision making and will require ongoing support and a 'safe space' in which she can discuss her fears and anxieties.

Using narrative therapy for abused women

The background to narrative therapies

Narrative therapies have their roots in the interdisciplinary (including social work) modernist theoretical approaches to family therapy. They have their epistemological roots in the sociological theories of Foucault (1980) and Goffman (1961; 1974), and in Bruner's (1986; 1990) and Bateson's (1972; 1979) studies of linguistics, text and meaning. The similarity of approaches within these narrative therapies, however, can tend to disguise their subtle differences of emphases.

The influence of Michael White

Amongst the many contributors to what can be described as this 'wide church' of narrative therapy, the names of Michael White (1989; 1995; 2000; 2007) and

David Epston (White and Epston, 1990) are cited by many writers as key contributors to the development of narrative approaches in therapy and social work. It will therefore be helpful to highlight some of their principal therapeutic concepts and techniques before discussing other approaches to narrative counselling and therapy:

> In striving to make sense of their lives, persons face the task of arranging their experiences of events in sequences across time in such a way as to arrive at a coherent account of themselves and the world around them.
>
> (White and Epston, 1990: 10)

Narrative, when used in this sense (as distinct from the literary sense), is a story-telling metaphor of the way we 'compose our lives' (Anderson, 1997). These stories or 'self-narratives' have 'emotional resonance', impacting not only on people's actions and attitudes, but also on their 'sense of identity'. They must have a beginning (i.e. history), a middle (i.e. present) and an end (i.e. future), and can therefore be future-determined as well as past-determined (White and Epston, 1990). In recounting these self-narratives, individuals often recount them in what White calls 'problem saturated talk', which gives life and support to the problem and the individual's or family's relationship with the problem. Stories are not merely a recounting of reality, they are themselves constitutive of reality.

'Recruiting an audience'

White (2007, 1995) and White and Epston (1990) have emphasised the importance of 'recruiting an audience' to witness to and authenticate the preferred stories of individuals in therapy. They utilise a range of techniques, including letters of invitation, awards and certificates, to involve this potential audience in what White (based on Myerhoff, 1982) describes as 'Definitional Ceremonies'. This enables the involvement of an audience who may or may not be actually physically present (or even still alive) to contribute to the consolidation of preferred identities and new meanings, as well as to the revision of previous meanings.

Narrative approaches to therapy and counselling reject the 'pathologising' power of expert knowledge and judgements and emphasise collaborative assessments of the causes of people's distress. Anderson (1997; 2007) specifically titles her work 'collaborative therapy'.

The contributions of narrative approaches to diversity and violence

The sensitivity to power relations in both the therapeutic relationship and in the wider social context is one of the important contributions of collaborative and narrative approaches.

Narrative process model

As noted in the previous section, narrative approaches are not a unitary phenomenon but are rather a family of therapeutic approaches whose influence on counselling and therapy is growing, and which are consequently themselves undergoing continual development (Payne, 2007). One such development is found in the work of Angus and colleagues (Angus *et al.*, 1999) who describe their approach as the Narrative Process Theory of therapy. The philosophical approach underpinning this theory or model of narrative therapy is indistinguishable from that of White and Epston or Anderson, as it is predicated on the assumption that successful psychotherapy entails the 'articulation, elaboration, and transformation of the client's self-told story or macronarrative'. Angus and her colleagues outline three distinct modes of inquiry within the therapeutic process: 1) The External Narrative Mode, which involves the description and elaboration of life events in the individual's life in which the story of 'what happened' is addressed; 2) The Internal Narrative Mode, which involves the exploration and elaboration of subjective feelings, reactions and emotions related to the events; and 3) the Reflexive Narrative Mode, which explores the meaning of both what happened and the emotions relating to it. The purpose of these processes is to develop a new understanding of 'what happened' which either supports or challenges the implicit beliefs which underpin the dominant narrative. According to Angus *et al.* (1999), this exploration of the subjective experience of events provides both worker and client with a 'rich spawning ground for the creation of new meanings'. This meaning making is facilitated by the exploration of personal expectations, needs and motivations, anticipations and beliefs of both the client and those individuals who play significant roles in the client's life.

As has been noted above, narrative approaches to social work and therapy are not a 'homogenous field'. Approaches differ epistemologically in their particular blend of modern and postmodern conceptualisations and practices (Brown and Augusta-Scott, 2007). Robert Neimeyer's therapeutic approach has grown explicitly out of a synthesis of social constructionism and constructivism, incorporating postmodern understandings of identity as a fluid, non essentialist, socially constructed 'saturated self' (Gergen, 1991) together with a contingent symbolic view of language as merely arbitrary 'signifiers' of meaning (Neimeyer, 1998).

Therapeutic approach

Starting from this philosophical (and political) stance, Neimeyer utilises the Narrative Process Model (NPM) of Angus *et al.* (1999) to develop his own therapeutic intervention approach. To this narrative process he adds a 'narrative structure' which includes setting, characterisation, plot, theme and fictional goal (Neimeyer and Levitt, 2001). The setting establishes the context of the story, the 'where and when' of the event(s). The characterisation refers to the 'who' of the story, the subjective worlds of the storyteller, and the other supporting characters. The plot is, as one would expect, the storyline of the events which fit together into a coherent account. The theme is the 'why', which provides a deeper level meaning which is often implicit and inferred. The fictional goal refers to the 'why' behind the plot. This is a term which is open to misunderstanding as it does not mean that the goal of the plot is untrue or imaginary. The term is drawn from the constructivist view and means that the self-narrative is 'fashioned or invented by the narrator' (Neimeyer and Levitt, 2001).

Neimeyer has developed a range of therapeutic techniques which can support distressed individuals in the disturbing challenge of rebuilding their world in the face of trauma and loss (Neimeyer, 2000). Amongst these techniques, the following would be suitable for working with abused women:

- biographies: a written record that provides an account of the significant events, persons, places and projects that shaped the individual's life;
- casual enactments: brief, informal roleplays designed to enable the individual to experiment with a particular part or role – these can also be non verbal;
- drawing and painting: symbolic drawings and artistic expressions can be interrogated for their nuances of meaning;
- journals: written narratives can enable individuals to confront and explore choices in relationships, place past traumas in a contemporary frame of reference and give 'voice' to unexpressed hopes;
- loss characterisations: open ended instructional prompts at the top of blank paper which gives an individual the opportunity to respond as they see fit, and which can then be interrogated for meaning in more formal ways;
- personal pilgrimage: to re-establish connections with persons, places and traditions that have grown distant or disconnected from our current lives.

This last technique would seem to be particularly appropriate for work with abused women for whom isolation from friends and family is a common form of control and abuse (Dobash and Dobash, 1998; Kirkwood, 1993).

Narrative social work in the context of abuse

Drawing on these approaches to, and interpretations of, narrative therapy and counselling, Wood and Roche (2001) and Roche and Wood (2005) explore the value of deconstructive narrative-based models of intervention. In their 2001 paper, 'An Emancipatory Principle for Social Work With Survivors of Male Violence', Wood and Roche note the need to 'repoliticize' interventions with abused women, which they claim has seen the theoretical base of such work overtaken by 'medical–psychological' approaches. Working from the premise of 'internalized oppression', they adapt the narrative approach of White (1989; 1995) and White and Epston (1990), to propose four transformative processes on which to base their model of intervention: (a) externalising; (b) deconstructive questioning; (c) seeking resistance-defiance; and (d) anchoring.

Transformative processes

The concept of 'externalising' is a widely accepted narrative therapy technique which separates the person from the problem. Rather than referring to the client's depression, the worker refers to '*the depression*' (Wood and Roche, 2001: 72). The risks involved in using externalising in the context of violence and abuse have been discussed earlier in this chapter. 'Deconstructive questioning' moves the narrative to a more political level, and helps the survivor to connect her personal experiences to wider cultural beliefs about women. These questions are informed by postmodern critiques of discourses, which identify and query the dominance of such discourses at both the personal and political levels. As Wood and Roche note, such awareness raising about the relationship of micro-level intimate abuse and wider oppressive cultural and gender discourses enables women to free themselves from self-blame, and may even encourage them to become involved at a more collective level in challenging such discourses and behaviours. They name the third process as 'Seeking resistance and defiance'. Their outline of this process resembles very closely the work of Alan Wade (1997; 2007), which has been discussed above. They affirm strongly that 'women *do* resist', and that 'this resistance takes many forms'. Their suggestion, however, is that 'searching for remembered moments . . . which foreshadow new stories of who the survivor is' (Wood and Roche, 2001: 76) links the concept of resistance with that of identity, which is the explicit purpose of the fourth process of this model. 'Anchoring' embeds the resistance of the present experience in the past. It suggests that the woman's current behaviour is rooted to some extent in her behaviour in the past. This concept resonates with Neimeyer and Levitt's (2001: 54) macro-narratives of resilience and coping.

In a later paper, Roche and Wood (2005) again suggest that their model of working with survivors of abuse starts from the need to counteract and challenge the pervasive 'woman blaming' that surrounds male violence against women, which they say is expressed by both perpetrators and those who purport to assist women. Their amended model, which they claim now contains three narrative processes for feminist social work, enables women to 'co-construct new identity stories' for themselves. They base their understanding of identity and resistance on the social constructionism of Berger and Luckmann (1967) and suggest that the necessary social work and counselling processes must also understand and engage identity as mutable and socially produced. They propose three interrelated processes in order to do this: (a) seeking resistance; (b) anchoring resistance; and (c) elaborating new stories. Seeking resistance in this model more closely resembles Wade's (1997; 2007) approach as it involves 'focused listening'.

Working with identity, meaning and resistance

Safety and crisis resolution may, however, initially be the woman's major concern, particularly if this encounter is her first attempt to seek professional help.

For the purposes of clarity, the intervention approach will be presented in three separate stages. Within these stages, the interrelationship of identity, meaning and resistance will be highlighted and clarified.

Stage 1: Safety first (versus safety only)

Finding resistance

The important concept of resistance (discussed in more detail in Chapter 4) high-lights the range of resistant responses in which women have engaged to protect both themselves and their children from increasing patterns of abuse. The first point of contact, therefore, with a professional social worker must recognise and honour these complex processes. Awareness of these processes must take equal precedence with an awareness of and concern for the physical safety of the woman and her children. Fears for a woman's safety tend to dominate early professional interventions, and this is entirely appropriate. It becomes inappropriate, however, when these concerns overwhelm and silence the voice of resistance and agency; 'safety first' can easily become 'safety only', leading to further oppression of a woman who has developed a myriad of survival and resistance skills. By focusing only on immediate physical safety, practitioners may enforce their own layer of control, justifying it on concerns about either the woman's or (more likely) the children's physical safety. The first task of this social work intervention, therefore, is to hold and acknowledge both these aspects of the woman's experience.

Narrating resistance

Taking cognisance of the risks to a woman's safety, particularly at the time of seeking external help or negotiating a change in the power dynamics of an abusive relationship, this intervention approach will begin with the voice and therefore the concerns of the abused woman. Appropriate and helpful questions at this point will be broad open questions, for example:

* 'Can you tell me what has been happening for you?'
* 'How you have been managing the situation up to now?'
* 'What have you been doing to keep yourself safe?'
* 'How has that worked for you?'
* 'What has changed recently?'
* 'What would you need to feel safer from now on?'

Questions such as these are examples of what can be described as 'open invitations to begin her narrative'. They help to create a space and dynamic in this particular professional relationship which will enable the abused woman to feel she can articulate her own voice. They are questions which enable the woman to narrate the 'external narrative' of her experience. Within that voice there will be clear indications of the levels of danger and risk to both herself and her children, as well as the strategies of resistance and safety seeking at which she will be adept, but which she may not fully appreciate. It is necessary for the social worker to bear in mind that most abused women will have spent years honing these resistance strategies, either years when they may have maintained a total silence about the abuse, or if it was known to her family or friends, years attempting to justify the relationship and perhaps even the partner's behaviour.

Recruiting an audience

The technique of recruiting an audience (White, 2007) of those who would have seen these resistances can help to surface and honour them at this point in the intervention. Questions which would be appropriate in recruiting this audience might be:

- 'Who saw you as stubborn (hard working/"mouthy") etc?'
- 'Who saw you stand up for yourself?'
- 'Who saw you challenge him on that occasion?'
- 'What would they say to you about that?'
- 'How would that help you to respond to his abuse?'
- 'What would they say to you now about your relationship with him?'

As she may not have heard support and appreciation for these strategies from informal or formal external sources, this recruited 'audience' can help to validate her narratives of resistance. Such validation of her 'small acts of daily living', to borrow the term Wade (1997) borrowed from Goffman (1961), focuses the conversation on the next steps to safety and survival.

Barriers to finding resistance

At this point of the intervention, questions which focus narrowly on children's safety, ignoring their mother's ingenuity and courage in protecting them from violence, will counteract the effectiveness of this 'open invitation' and influence a narrow and defensive narrative – echoing the dominant discourses of the responsibilities of motherhood which have led to the 'mixed' outcomes of social work with abused women in child protection settings. Women are rarely if ever unaware of the risks to their children from abusive partners.

Other resources

Intervention at this early stage may also involve referral to a women's refuge or other place of safety, either on a temporary or semi permanent basis. It will probably involve advice regarding the legal options open to a woman, such as a Safety or a Barring Order. It may involve referral to a Legal Aid solicitor, or to the court accompaniment service of a specialised domestic violence service.

Going further (and deeper)

Finding meaning and identity

Once the immediate danger to the woman (and/or her children) has been assessed and appropriate strategies to increase her safety have been negotiated and implemented by her and with her, the next stage of this intervention model can be given greater emphasis. (It is important to keep in mind that safety is not a 'once off' achievement. The woman and the social worker may need to return to the issues of safety, legal processes and accommodation a number of times.)

Questions influenced by the Narrative Process Theory (Angus *et al.*, 1999) can help to find and narrate these meanings. External narrative questions enable the opening up of the intervention process. Internal and reflexive narrative questions can now enable the exploration of meaning:

- 'What were your hopes for the relationship when you married (moved in) with your partner/husband?' (Internal Narrative)
- 'How did you imagine it would work out?' (Internal Narrative)
- 'What did your family/friends think about your relationship?' (Reflexive Narrative)
- 'What did you begin to think when the abuse/control began?' (Internal Narrative)
- 'How did your partner/husband explain his behaviour?' (Internal Narrative)
- 'Did that make sense to you?' (Reflexive Narrative)
- 'Where do you think he got those ideas?' (Reflexive Narrative)
- 'Who else in your community/family held those kinds of ideas?' (Reflexive Narrative)
- 'Where do you think they came from?' (Reflexive Narrative)

This narrative process will also enable her to recognise the manner in which she resisted these discourses at the local level – and in doing so, how she resisted the imposition of the unwanted identity of the 'battered woman'. Questions which may help with this narrating of her identity would be:

- 'How would you describe the (young) woman who began this relationship?'
- 'How did you see yourself when the abuse began?'
- 'How did you see yourself as you did (example of resistance) to protect yourself?'
- 'How do you see yourself now that the relationship is ending/over?'
- 'How would you describe the woman who has got to this point?'

All of these processes will clearly not occur in one session, and, as discussed above, may be interspersed with the practicalities of legal, housing or safety concerns. While these counselling and practical issues may be separated conceptually, they are of course not separate in reality. They are all part of the journey to safety, but, as with any complicated and challenging journey where the precise destination is not known, there will need to be constant checking and rechecking of the goals of the journey, the possible choice of roads that can be taken, the areas that are best bypassed and the ones that need to be visited. For this reason, the map may need to be redrawn on a regular basis, depending on the exigencies of external circumstances (e.g. children's schooling needs, economic necessity, illness, increased partner violence, insufficient police support). Within this uncertainty of destination and navigation, however, the counselling process will continue to elucidate and foreground the woman's preferred identity, her meaning construction of the relationship, the meaning of intimacy, the meaning of abuse and control, and the relationship of her strategies of resistance (small as they may seem to her) to these constructions of meaning and evolving identity. This process leads to the co-construction of the woman's new meanings and preferred identity.

Safety proofing

The third stage of this intervention approach can be described as 'safety proofing' for the woman's future. It is sometimes assumed that once a woman takes a legal order (e.g. a Protection or a Barring Order) or moves to a refuge, the social worker's or support person's job is done. She (and her children) are now safe. This is the risk of 'safety first' becoming 'safety only'. What others may see as the ultimate success of their interventions is, for the woman, just the first step on a long, difficult and life changing journey. If she is left without ongoing support at this point of making life changing decisions, she may find that she is unable to take herself to an unknown destination without a road map and/or apparent means of getting there. It is at this point that long-term decisions will need to be made. A range of narrative style questions which will be helpful at this stage, and which foreground her preferred identity, are:

- 'How would you describe yourself at this point?' (Identity question)
- 'Is this the woman you wanted to be when you got married?' (Preferred Identity question)
- 'Who do you want to be in the future?' (Preferred Identity question)
- 'What are you doing to become this woman?' (Action question)
- 'Who can help you in this?' (Resourcing question)
- 'What would they say to (or do for) you now?' (Witness question)
- 'If you take this step, what will they say about you?' (Witness question)
- 'Who will you be if you do this?' (Preferred Identity question).

Survival resistance

As with her experience of surviving an abusive relationship, her post separation experiences will also involve what has been identified as 'survival resistance'. This may involve legal battles for access to and custody of children, or the transfer and ownership of property. It may involve getting a new job, taking up educational opportunities, becoming a single parent to possibly angry and traumatised children, or moving to a new neighbourhood. It will require ongoing reconstruction of the meaning of these experiences, similar to that for those who are bereaved, but with the added grief of disappointment, regret and possibly ongoing fear. Narrative techniques, such as transition ceremonies, diaries and journals may be helpful in marking and, where possible, celebrating the stages of the journey which have been reached, and their meaning in the overall goal of co-constructing her preferred future with a preferred, now clearly evolving identity. This identity will be informed by both a woman's previous identity and by her experiences of surviving, and increasingly, thriving. (For further information on this approach to counselling abused women, see Allen, 2012b.)

Support groups

As well as individual counselling techniques (such as narrative therapy approaches discussed above), support groups for abused women can also be extremely supportive for women and children. Such support groups – based on the principles of building self-esteem, self-determination and empowerment – have proved an important addition to the range of support services provided by specialised women's voluntary organisations and social workers. Support groups include at least three types of formal and informal structures:

1   groups completely self-managed by survivors, who may or may not have accessed existing domestic violence services;
2   informal groups – facilitated by staff and/or volunteers with experience of working with survivors;
3   formal group programmes – such as Pattern Changing for Abused Women: An Educational Program, or the Freedom Programme in the UK – also facilitated by staff and/or volunteers with experience of working with survivors and a thorough knowledge of the effects of domestic violence on women and children.

Information from: http://www.freedomprogramme.co.uk/
freedomprogramme/index.cfm34

Domestic abuse, in the long run, erodes self-esteem and social skills, destroys family intimacy, damages growing children, reduces parenting skills and creates intense feelings of shame, guilt, isolation and loneliness. In stark contrast to abuse, support groups lessen isolation and establish social bonds. Sharing life stories can combat feelings of shame and guilt; women can find help and learn coping strategies, for example for dealing with their traumatised children, while at the same time they lessen their sense of inadequacy (*The Power To Change*, 2008).

Conclusion

This chapter has outlined the range of activities that a social worker (or other professional) needs to engage in when working with an abused woman. Safety planning, knowledge of the legal processes in each country, awareness of local helplines and refuges, their phone numbers and addresses are all essential information the worker must have. Individual counselling of the woman, using narrative therapy as described above, is a very helpful approach to take with supporting abused women, keeping in mind their resistance, identity and meaning. Support groups are also very helpful and can provide women with an understanding of the range of abuse they have been experiencing and can provide them with empowerment skills. This range of activities is essential to support women dealing with or leaving an abusive relationship, and involves skills that every social worker should have when working with abused women.

6   Interventions in a medical, midwifery and mental health setting

Social workers, nurses, midwives and doctors working in hospitals and mental health settings encounter the effects of intimate partner violence on a daily basis. As the World Health Organization (WHO) has pointed out, health professionals and social workers in hospitals frequently, and often unknowingly, come into contact with women affected by abuse, as they make extensive use of health care services (WHO, 2010). Intimate partner violence has long-term negative health consequences for survivors, even after the abuse has ended (Campbell, 2002: 1331). Being able to recognise such abuse, intervene appropriately and provide appropriate support and information to abused women is an essential aspect of good practice in this context. There is a range of studies which outline the risk to women of intimate partner abuse, and these will be reviewed. Appropriate intervention strategies will also be discussed in this chapter and the range of information and strategies that should be undertaken to assist abused women will be outlined.

Effects of abuse on women victims

'Battering by a partner is the single major cause of injury to women in the USA. It is the single biggest reason women are admitted to casualty units' (*Mental Health: A Report of the Surgeon General*, 1999). In addition to being a breach of human rights, intimate partner violence is associated with serious public health consequences (Ellsberg *et al.*, 2008).

In the past decade, increasing attention has been focused on the effects of male partner violence on women's physical and mental health. Studies of visits to emergency departments in the USA and elsewhere have suggested that physical abuse is a major cause of injury in women. Population-based studies have suggested that 20–75% of women who are physically abused by a partner report injuries due to violence at some point in their lives. Nonetheless, injury is not the most common physical health outcome of abuse by male partners. Epidemiological and clinical studies have noted that physically and sexually violent acts by intimate partners are consistently associated with a broad array of negative health outcomes, including gynaecological disorders, adverse pregnancy outcomes, irritable bowel syndrome, gastrointestinal disorders, and various chronic pain syndromes. Abused women have more physical symptoms of poor health, and more days in bed, than do women who have not been abused. Physical and sexual violence have also been associated with psychiatric problems, including depression, anxiety, phobias, post-traumatic stress disorder (PTSD), suicidality, and alcohol and drug abuse.

Research on the health effects of intimate partner violence has been constrained by several factors. Most studies have been undertaken on clinical rather than population-based samples, mainly in North America and Europe. Furthermore, many studies have had small sample sizes, and have not controlled analyses for potential confounders. Violence has not been defined or measured consistently in the studies, making comparisons difficult.

A study carried out in the USA (Macy *et al.*, 2009) reviewed a range of studies that explored women's physical and mental health conditions that social workers are likely to see in their practices. They reviewed 3,500 research articles, which were all peer reviewed and examined the impact of partner violence on women's physical and mental health outcomes. Amongst the findings of this review the outcomes for women experiencing intimate partner violence were very clear. For example, Carbonne-Lopez *et al.* (2006) in a national representative survey of 5,991 women found that, compared to women who said they were not abused (77% of the sample), women who experienced interpersonal conflict had higher rates of poor self-reported health, injury disability, depression, mental health disability, tranquilliser and sedative use, antidepressant use, prescription pain pill use and recreational drug use. In a study by Carlson *et al.* (2002) of women attending primary care centres, 14% reported physical aggression in the past year, 46.1% reported emotional abuse, and 5.7% reported forced sex in the past year, and reported high levels of depression and anxiety. In a study by Coker *et al.* (2000) in family medical practice clinics, of which 53.6% of participants reported partner violence in their lifetimes, psychological violence was related to poor physical and mental health, and physical violence was also related to poor physical and mental health, with women attending their GP on five occasions in the past year. Having ever experienced physical partner abuse was associated with increased risk of hearing loss, angina, heart/circulatory problems, bladder and kidney infections, hysterectomy and gastric reflux. In a study by Tolman and Wang (2005), they found that partner violence affects women's ability to work by negatively affecting their physical and mental health. Summarising these findings, Macy *et al.* (2009) concluded that these datasets demonstrate that partner violence and its negative effects on women's physical and mental health, including drug and alcohol use, are widespread problems among women of all ages, sociocultural backgrounds and socioeconomic groups. As the severity of partner abuse increased, women reported increasingly severe health consequences in a predictable way. Women who reported abuse in their childhood, as well as partner abuse as adults, reported more health problems. This demonstrates that repeat victimisation over the course of a woman's lifetime can also seriously undermine her health. Amongst violence survivors, chronic pain disorders include back and neck pain, migraines and headaches, pelvic pain and arthritis. Survivors also experience a variety of gastrointestinal disorders, including stomach ulcers, spastic colon, gastric reflux, indigestion and diarrhoea (Campbell, 2002).

Mental health outcomes include depression, anxiety, PTSD and suicidal ideation and attempts. Some research has shown that survivors of violence are likely to have co-occurring mental illness such as depression and PTSD. There is also a relationship between drug and alcohol abuse and intimate partner violence. Abuse survivors also use the health services and mental health services more than other women. Unfortunately, many women do not identify themselves as abuse survivors or as currently experiencing abuse, which leads to the need for screening and sensitive questioning.

In a review of US and Canadian studies, Campbell (2002) reports that gynaecological problems are the most consistent and long-lasting effects for abused women experiencing forced sex as opposed to non-abused women. Differential symptoms and conditions include sexually transmitted diseases, vaginal bleeding or infection, fibroids, decreased sexual desire, genital irritation, pain on intercourse, chronic pelvic pain and urinary tract infections (Campbell, 2002: 1332). As Campbell (2002) points out, abused women are likely to use health care services at least three times more than non-abused women. In another study she cites, battered women are likely to generate around 92% more health costs per year than non battered women, with mental health services accounting for most of the increased costs (Wisner *et al.*, 1999). Campbell suggests that as women are more likely to use health care settings before reporting to the criminal justice or social services, routine screening should be carried out in all health care settings.

In a Swedish study (Linton, 2002), a random sample of participants between the ages of 35 and 45, 449 reported no pain, 229 reported mild pain and 271 reported pronounced pain. For these women the risk of pronounced pain increased fivefold in those who experienced physical abuse and fourfold for those who experienced sexual abuse. These forms of abuse were associated with the development of acute onset back pain as well as functional impairment.

In a study by Humphreys and Absler (2011) in the USA, they explored the extent of chronic pain in a community sample. Responses to their request for participants were received by 84 women, ranging in age from 19 to 76 years. Of these women, 59% were abused by their boyfriends, while 39% were abused by their husbands. Pain longer than three months in duration was reported by 77% of the participants. Of the 65 women who reported chronic pain, 25% were categorised in the mild pain group while 75% were in the moderate to severe pain group. Women in the latter category were less likely to be employed and were in an abusive relationship longer than the women with mild chronic pain. These women also described their pain as 'miserable' (74%) 'sharp' (63%) and 'unbearable' (49%). The majority of women in the mild and moderate to severe categories experienced psychological aggression, sexual coercion, physical assault and injuries from abuse. Women in the moderate to severe group were more likely to report minor injuries and threats of physical violence than were women in the mild chronic pain group. These figures are much higher than prevalence reported of chronic pain in Western country population samples (Humphreys *et al.*,

2011: 1337). In fact these mean scores are comparable with people with arthritis or metastatic cancer. Humphreys *et al.* (2011: 1338) conclude that 'when multiple physical and psychological stressors like those associated with IPV [intimate partner violence] activate stress-regulation systems, the result can overwhelm the body and create patterns that result in chronic pain'.

WHO multi-country study

The aim of the WHO multi-country study (Ellsberg *et al.*, 2008) was to explore the magnitude and characteristics of different forms of physical, sexual and emotional violence against women, with particular emphasis on violence perpetrated by male intimate partners. The study attempted to overcome obstacles of comparability encountered in previous studies by use of population-based surveys that included a standardised questionnaire, and with standardised training and data collection across participating sites. A further objective of the study was to assess the extent to which physical and sexual violence by intimate partners is associated with a range of health outcomes. This report presents findings on partner violence and women's self-reported physical and mental health.

The analysis of all sites found significant associations between lifetime experiences of partner violence and self-reported poor health, and with specific health problems in the previous four weeks, which included difficulty walking, difficulty with daily activities, pain, memory loss, dizziness, and vaginal discharge. For all settings combined, women who reported partner violence at least once in their life reported significantly more emotional distress, suicidal thoughts and suicidal attempts than non-abused women. These significant associations were maintained in almost all of the sites. Between 19% and 55% of women who had ever been physically abused by their partner were injured (Ellsberg *et al.*, 2008).

Intimate partner violence also exerts serious socioeconomic effects on women. As financial abuse and control is often an integral part of intimate partner violence, abused women may not have access to their own income, even if they are working outside the home. They may not be allowed to drive the family car, or visit friends and relatives. Moving house to ensure that neighbours and friends do not become involved in the support of the woman also means that she is socially isolated and does not know whom to trust. As she may also be constantly told that she is stupid and does not know how to raise her children, she will lose her self-confidence and develop very poor self-esteem. The effects of these forms of emotional and financial abuse will help to undermine her ability to take action to protect herself. *Fear* is the one of the most consistent effects of serious abuse (Allen and Perttu, 2010).

Violence in pregnancy

According to the WHO, most studies of abuse during pregnancy measure only physical violence. However, as they point out, sexual and emotional abuse during pregnancy are also considered as detrimental for women's and their children's wellbeing (WHO, 2011). International figures on the abuse of pregnant women suggest that 1% of pregnant women in Japan and 28% in Peru experience abuse during pregnancy, with the average ranging from 4% to 12% (Garcia-Moreno *et al.*, 2005). A study by Campbell *et al.* (2004) found that women in Egypt are assaulted at a rate of 32% during pregnancy, followed by India with a rate of 28%, 21% in Saudi Arabia and 11% in Mexico. A recent study in Africa found rates of 23–40% for physical abuse, 3–27% for sexual abuse and 25–49% for emotional abuse during pregnancy. The consequences of such abuse can have both fatal and non fatal adverse health outcomes for pregnant women and their children due to the trauma of abuse to the woman's body, as well as the physiological effects of stress from current or past abuse on fetal growth and development. A US study found that pregnancy significantly increases a woman's risk of becoming a victim of intimate partner femicide, and that men who abuse their pregnant partners seem to be very dangerous and more likely to commit homicide (Campbell *et al.*, 2003).

Non fatal outcomes during pregnancy include maternal and new born health outcomes. Some research has shown that women reporting abuse during pregnancy had higher rates of intrauterine growth retardation and preterm labour than women not experiencing abuse. It has also been associated with increased risk of miscarriage and abortion. Intimate partner violence during pregnancy is also associated with a number of adverse health behaviours such as smoking, alcohol and drug use, in order to cope with the stress, shame and suffering caused by the abuse (Campbell, 2002). Injuries can also include broken bones, cuts, burns, haemorrhages, broken teeth and persistent headaches. Direct blows to the abdomen can cause the negative reproductive health outcomes outlined in Figure 6.1.

There is no clear research which clarifies whether physical abuse begins during pregnancy or is just a continuation of previous abuse. The WHO study (Garcia-Moreno *et al.*, 2005) found that 50% of the women in three sites were beaten for the first time during pregnancy. Campbell *et al.* (1993) suggest that violence during pregnancy followed four themes: 1) jealousy towards the future child; 2) pregnancy-specific violence not directed towards the foetus; 3) anger towards the foetus; and 4) 'business as usual' where violence continues in the same manner as before pregnancy. A more recent study by Graham-Kevan and Archer (2011) found that 47% of a sample of battered women had experienced abuse during pregnancy. Abdominal blows during their pregnancies were reported by 65% of the participants. They also reported more control, involving isolation from family and friends, than did women who were not struck on the abdomen. The authors found that these women were younger and had been in their relationships for a shorter time. They concluded that the abusive partner suspected that the child might not be his. His anger could also be directed at the changes to the woman during pregnancy, such as a reduction in sexual activity. In terms of emotional jealousy, the woman's affection for a new third party – the baby – might also motivate his jealousy. The authors suggest that further research is required to test these hypotheses.

In a quantitative Swedish study, Edin *et al.* (2010) explored the reasons why women did not tell midwives when attending antenatal clinics about the violence

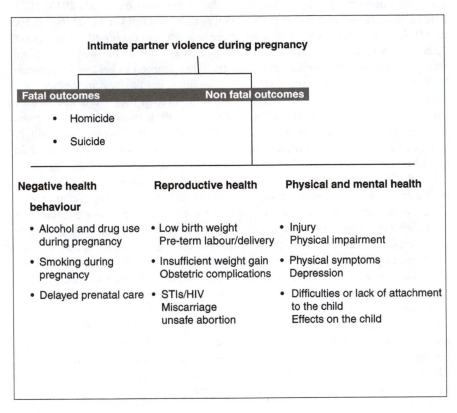

Figure 6.1 Intimate partner violence during pregnancy.

Source: WHO, 2011

they were experiencing. All nine of the women in the study had experienced severe physical and/or sexual violence and/or threats of brutal violence during at least one pregnancy. They were all well educated and were in employment. All of the women had left their partners when the child was a baby or a little older. The descriptions of violence included all kinds of brutality and three women had been kicked in the abdomen or been jumped on, on the abdomen. They also felt that their partners' behaviour changed for the worse during their pregnancy. The women described that their partners controlled and oppressed them as if they owned both them and their pregnancies. The women felt frightened and stressed during the pregnancy. As one woman described it: 'It is not good for someone who is pregnant to land on the floor, backwards, or have his weight on you. And you see, I was dead scared' (Edin *et al*., 2010: 193). Another woman described the trigger that started the abuse when she was six months pregnant: 'I did not do the dishes, when he thought I should do them or such, it was not such big things but very small matters, then he kicked me in the stomach' (Edin *et al.*, 2010: 193). One partner refused to travel in the car with her: 'he did not want a fat toad in the car' (Edin *et al.*, 2010: 194). However, these women also exercised resistance (as discussed in Chapter 4). The women learned to get out of the way – to avoid further violence to themselves or their baby. They learned to behave in a certain way so as not to give free rein to their personalities, but to obey unquestionably. However, they did not hold back all of the time, even if they were scared: they said no to sex, were critical and obstinate, made their own decisions, showed anger and argued back (Edin *et al.*, 2010: 194). All but one woman increasingly questioned their relationships, and most planned to leave, when it was safe to do so. Some of the men never left their partner's side at the prenatal clinic, which raises the issue again of providing the woman with personal space to speak alone with a professional. However, even though three of the women told the midwives what was occurring at home, only one found a sympathetic response. Screening is not routine in Swedish prenatal clinics. Many of the women did not tell anyone as they 'felt it would be too demanding to let someone else into their situation when all their energy was absorbed in putting up with life in general' (Edin *et al.*, 2010: 197). The women described 'feelings of shame, lack of confidence in the midwives, seeing them as authorities' and viewing the prenatal visits as threatening events. The authors suggest that a short screening question such as a routine question when taking the patients' history would be helpful to identify abuse. However, they feel that the outcome of this question or screening is dependent on the communication in the encounter, such as how the needs of the women are met. This brings us back to the need to respect women's decisions, providing them with information on services, refuges and legal options without demanding that they do what we want them to do. Replacing one form of control with another form is not what abused women need or want.

The study by Lipsky *et al.* (2004) in the USA concludes that screening of pregnant women is a critical issue in antenatal care. They particularly mention women hospitalised because of substance abuse or with mental health problems, which as has been seen are defensive mechanisms and outcomes which abused women experience. The American College of Obstetricians and Gynaecologists and the American Medical Association recommend routine intimate partner violence screening for all patients. Meuleners *et al.* (2011) also suggest education for younger pregnant women on the impact of intimate partner violence. Such programmes can be incorporated into prenatal education programmes, and may also help younger women to disclose such abuse and avail of social work help within the maternity hospital.

Mental health settings

Exposure to partner violence can lead to prolonged mental health disorders, and even suicidality. The most prevalent mental health sequelae which abused women present with are depression, anxiety, substance use and PTSD. As outlined by Hegarty and O'Doherty (2011), these psychological indicators of partner abuse are as follows:

- insomnia
- depression
- suicidal ideation
- anxiety symptoms and panic disorder
- somatoform disorder
- post-traumatic stress disorder
- eating disorders
- drug and alcohol abuse.

In a Spanish study Pico-Alfonso (2005) points out that PTSD is the most frequent mental health consequence of intimate partner violence, with a mean prevalence of 64% in abused women. Characteristic features of PTSD include re-experiencing the traumatic event, emotional numbness or avoidance and increased arousal. Cascardi *et al.* (1999) reviewed a number of studies which found that PTSD amongst abused women ranged from 31% to 84% with modal rates ranging between 45% and 60%. Their study involved 127 women with a mean age of 44.16 years. In this group they found that women who were physically abused were also psychologically abused and 32% were also sexually abused. Their study found that the main predictor of PTSD was intimate partner violence. Women experiencing intimate partner violence had a significantly higher rate of PTSD as compared to the control group. They found that 80.1% of the intimate partner violence victims reported that their PTSD was abuse related. The degree of psychological abuse (intimation, coercive control) appears to be a stronger indicator of fear within intimate partner violence than the severity of physical abuse and leads to higher levels of PTSD and depression. When they separated the psychological, physical and sexual violence they found that the psychological component turned out to the strongest indicator, followed by sexual and physical abuse. They found no significant difference in the PTSD symptoms of women who had left their partners in the previous 12 months.

In a US study, Carbonne-Lopez *et al.* (2006) also explored the relationship between substance use and mental health difficulties in women experiencing intimate partner violence. Women who are regularly abused are three times as likely to experience severe depression and other forms of mental disorders than non-abused women and four times as likely to report a mental health disability. They are also more likely to report drinking alcohol every day than women who are not abused (Carbonne-Lopez *et al.*, 2000: 390). The authors also found elevated rates of using tranquillisers, sleeping pills, sedatives, antidepressants and recreational drugs. As a result of their findings, they encourage the use of screening tools in clinical mental health settings.

In a number of other studies, PTSD was found in 33–83% of battered women, and is the most frequent mental disorder in this population (Bargai *et al.*, 2007). Previous abuse as a child can also increase a woman's likelihood of experiencing PTSD if she is abused as an adult. In a study carried out by Bargai *et al.* (2007), they explored the relationship between learned helplessness, which results from repeated exposure to uncontrollable and aversive events. Domestic abuse clearly falls in this category. They used the Beck Depression Inventory and the Structured Clinical Interview for DSM-IV [Diagnostic and Statistical Manual of Mental Disorders]. Their study confirmed previous studies which found a significant overlap of PTSD and depression in abused women, and a significant occurrence of the two together (Bargai *et al.*, 2007: 273). They also found that learned helplessness magnifies the pathogenic effect of such abuse. They concluded that in abused women, higher scores of PTSD are associated with higher scores for learned helplessness. They also found that learned helplessness was associated with biographical factors, particularly with a male dominated background:

> In other words, educational and cultural influences which promote female submissiveness and prejudice against women are most likely undermining the emotional resources and coping skills of women who grow up in such environments, thereby increasing their likelihood of developing PTSD and depression as a consequence of male violence.
>
> (Bargai *et al.*, 2007: 273)

Child abuse was also significantly associated with learned helplessness, PTSD and depression. Even amongst women who leave abusive relationships, they also found that there is still a high level of PTSD and depression. It therefore cannot be assumed that once a woman has left a violent relationship, these symptoms will all disappear. The authors suggest that empowerment interventions may greatly help women to combat learned helplessness and depression and these are strategies which social workers in mental health settings should seriously consider.

In a well-known study by Stark and Flitcraft (1996), they traced 176 women who were admitted to hospital as a result of an attempted suicide who had previously presented with intimate partner violence in a general hospital. Of these 176 participants, 29.5% were battered women. Of these women, 22.2% had at least one incident of domestic abuse in their records, and 7.3% had at least one injury that resulted from an assault. The remaining 70.4% of the women were not believed to have experienced domestic abuse. Of those abused, 85% had made at least one visit to the general hospital as a result of an assault. On the same day as their suicide attempt, 36.5% of the women visited the hospital with an injury attributable to abuse. Abused women who attempted suicide also did so more frequently than non-abused women. Of the abused women 21.1% had attempted suicide three times or more. This compares with 8% of the women who were not abused. Stark and Flitcraft also found that the abuse was very rarely selected as the focus of the intervention. Of the non-abused women 94% were referred to a mental health service, whereas 22% of the abused women did not elicit a referral to a mental health facility or a social service of any kind. This study shows that both general hospitals and mental health facilities need to take into account the possibility that a woman's suicide attempt is related to intimate partner violence and that the use of a screening instrument is important in assessing such incidents.

WHO recommendations for dealing with abuse in medical settings

The WHO (2010) has made a number of suggestions for the identification of abused women and the education of staff to recognise and deal with such abuse. They suggest that the identification of abused women can range from screening all pregnant women to selective screening. Selective screening can be initiated through the identification of women with depression, anxiety or repeat sexually transmitted infections. Once women are identified as abused, careful documentation is necessary. Photographs can provide compelling evidence if cases come to court. In some countries (such as Ireland), women may take their midwifery notes home with them. In such cases, recording abuse in these notes would increase the likelihood of further abuse by her partner. Alternative means of keeping such records would need to be developed. For example, once a woman has been identified as being abused, the social worker should become involved and these records and photographs can be held in the social worker's case notes.

Training

The WHO emphasises the need to train medical personnel in all medical settings to recognise and deal with intimate partner violence. They suggest that all personnel should be given awareness raising sessions to sensitise them to the issue. They should be trained in how to listen to women and how to ask about partner violence and how to support and validate disclosure, documentation and record keeping. (Once a woman discloses abuse she should be referred to the medical social worker, who is skilled in dealing with such sensitive issues, and who should inform the woman of her rights, provide her with support and information, and keep in touch with her in a safe and confidential manner.) The WHO also suggests training between health care organisations and external agencies in order to facilitate the referral process and promote an understanding of what kinds of support different organisations can provide. This is currently happening in Ireland, where the Women's Aid Training Department is working with mental health and maternity hospitals to help them establish screening tools, and educate the staff on the complex issues of intimate partner violence.

WHO responses to violence against women

The WHO (2010) has also published a document which makes suggestions for the enhancement of services to women within health services across the world. They outline the range of issues that need to be addressed within this sector:

how to ensure that the response becomes institutionalized (i.e. changing individual behaviour and organizational culture); how to maintain multisectoral collaboration and collaboration with women's nongovernmental organizations (NGOs); how to ensure that women are not placed at further risk by any intervention; the range of forms of violence it is realistic to address in different health-care settings; which health-care settings are most appropriate for offering these services; should there be routine screening for partner violence or more selective enquiry for improved clinical management; and what are the key lessons about provider training in terms of minimum content and duration (2010: 1).

They quote the Ramsay *et al.* (2005) review which outlines that advocacy interventions can reduce the levels of abuse, increase social support and quality of life and lead to increased use of safety behaviours and accessing of community resources.

The WHO also states that there is sufficient evidence to suggest that screening for partner violence is acceptable to women. Health professionals should be trained to ask directly about partner violence when women present with certain conditions, such as injuries; symptoms of anxiety, depression or substance abuse; sexually transmitted infections; repeat non-specific symptoms; recurrent gynaecological symptoms; and during the course of antenatal/prenatal care. The way the questions are asked is important, as it can discourage women (e.g. 'You're not a victim of domestic violence, are you?'). Screening tools have been developed and tested and, coupled with training in how to ask, they have been shown to increase the identification of women suffering violence.

Studies show that what women want from health-care providers is:

- before disclosure or questioning: to try and ensure continuity of care;
- to make it possible for women to disclose current and past abuse;
- when the issue of partner violence is raised, not to pressurise women to fully disclose;
- that the immediate response to disclosure is to ensure that women feel they have control over the situation and to address any safety issues;
- that in later consultations, the health-care provider should understand the chronic nature of the problem and provide follow-up support.

Recording and documenting

Recording injuries and disclosures of intimate partner violence is an important task for health and social work personnel for a number of reasons:

- These records may be necessary as evidence in a court case, if a woman seeks a civil protection order or if her partner is charged in the criminal system.
- They may be necessary if there are legal proceedings regarding custody of and access to children if the couple separate.

- Having a record within the hospital system ensures that future injures (or death) are examined with the possibility of intimate partner violence in mind.
- Keeping a record of attendance at a clinic can provide a red flag regarding escalating risk.

However, the manner in which these records are kept must be in accordance with the principles of good practice.

Document the evidence – the nature and location of all injuries, new injuries and old injuries, use Body Maps, and use detailed verbal descriptions.

- Record a brief statement from the victim/patient regarding how she was injured and who caused her injuries.
- The name of the abuser and his relationship to the victim/patient should be recorded.
- Record time, date, and place of assault, and witnesses, if any.
- Record name and number of any police involved, details of weapons used, if any, details of any witnesses present.
- Record a brief statement from the victim/patient regarding the history of previous violence in the relationship.
- If injuries are not consistent with the statement given by victim/patient and if she maintains her position having being challenged the record should reflect this. The doctor should record that in his/her opinion the injuries are in inconsistent with the explanation given.
- Use non-judgemental terms in describing the patient's statement as to the cause of her injuries. Use phrases such as 'the patient says . . .'
- Avoid using terms such as 'the patient alleges' – such language sounds judgemental and implies the writer does not believe what the patient says.
- Document injuries with photographs – having obtained consent. Photographs must be taken with a Polaroid camera, or phone that takes pictures, and must be signed by the person who took them.
- Preserve any physical evidence.

Adapted from *Domestic Violence: A Health Issue:*
Guidelines for Hospital Staff, 2004

Case examples

The following examples from the medical, midwifery and mental health field can provide some guidance on how social workers (and other professionals in these settings) can identify abused women and provide them with support and intervention.

A young woman is admitted to the A & E Department with a severely bruised arm and pain in her back. This is the second time she has been admitted with bruising and pain. In view of the fact that this is not her first admission with such injuries, all the staff should be alert to the possibility of intimate partner abuse. Firstly her husband/partner should not be allowed to remain with her when the staff are enquiring about her injuries. (Women will not disclose abuse when their partners are present.) Staff need to be alert to the phenomenon of grooming by partners. This can mean the partner/husband is extremely charming to the staff, making it impossible for them to realise he is an abusive partner. Sometimes, when this charm offensive does not work, the partner can become very angry with staff, making them afraid and unwilling to continue with the holistic care of the woman. However, it is important that staff are aware that this grooming can occur, and are prepared to deal with this behaviour. Once the woman is on her own, and cannot be heard by her partner, staff need to ask her if anyone has abused her. (The *Mid-West Area Adult Mental Health Domestic Violence Assessment Tool*, 2005) may be useful here as it is not long, but can provide the woman with the opportunity to disclose abuse.) If the woman is very scared of her partner, she may be afraid to disclose domestic abuse. In this case, it is important that staff ask the medical social worker to talk to her, and s/he should give her the names of relevant agencies (such as Women's Aid, refuges, legal options etc.). The medical social worker should also give her the opportunity to return to the social worker if she wishes to discuss things further.

If the woman does disclose to the nursing staff, the medical staff or the medical social worker that she has been abused, the staff should immediately involve the social worker (if not already involved). Again, a clear discussion with the woman about the level of abuse, the fear the woman may be experiencing and her fears for her children (if she has children) needs to occur. Very few women will make a decision within the hospital setting about their future, but the medical social worker needs to offer her available options, such as access to a refuge, talking to the social worker in the near future, her legal options or referral to Women's Aid or some organisation with specialised knowledge of domestic violence. It is very important in all of these discussions that her husband is not aware of what is occurring between the woman and the staff. If he is aware, he will become more violent and more controlling to ensure she cannot talk to anyone else. As was seen in the WHO guidelines above, it is essential that all staff in direct contact with abused women are trained in the recognition of such abuse, are aware of the grooming that may occur, and are aware that speaking to both partners directly is very dangerous for the woman. In a case where an abused woman was admitted for an x-ray, she claimed (because her partner was with her all the time) that she fell down the stairs. When the x-ray results were reported to the doctor, he came to her bedside, where her husband was sitting, and told her that she could not have fallen down the stairs as the x-ray showed something quite different. Her husband was holding her hand, and as a result of the pressure he placed on her hand, so that she would not tell the doctor, he broke her hand also. If this doctor had been aware that he should not speak to both partners together, this further injury would not have occurred.

As was seen in the previous chapter, safety plans can be helpful for women. However, keeping phone numbers and other material about domestic violence in the house can leave the woman in further danger. If she has a friend nearby, with whom she can leave this material, this can be helpful. Sometimes women being treated by physiotherapists may disclose this abuse to this professional, and the physiotherapist needs to refer the patient to the medical social worker. Again, the training of all staff is important in a medical setting so that all know the danger signs, and to whom to refer the patient. The medical social worker may need to accompany the woman to the court to support her. S/he may refer the woman to a lawyer, but the woman may still need support in the courtroom. It is important for social workers to be fully cognisant of the legal options in their jurisdiction, as women will need accurate and timely information as to what their legal options are.

Midwifery setting

A young woman in her twenties is attending the antenatal service of her local maternity hospital. She got pregnant earlier than she and her partner had planned, and he blames her for this. Having completed the screening questionnaire, she discloses that her partner has hit her, and constantly controls and demeans her. She is terrified of being alone, given the forthcoming baby and her lack of employment. She is determined to stay with her partner. (See Kelly, 1995 and the phases of disengagement outlined on pp. 42–43.) The social worker is called to discuss this issue with her, when she discloses abuse to the nursing staff. The social worker respects her decision, but outlines that this form of violence may get worse. She works with the woman to draw up a safety plan (see Chapter 5). She is informed about her local refuge, and about Women's Aid helpline and their support services. The social worker offers to see this woman on a regular basis.

Once the baby is born her partner becomes even more violent. The woman now talks to the social worker about the option of leaving. She is terrified for her own wellbeing and that of her baby, but she will not go to a refuge. The social worker suggests she take out a Barring Order against her partner. S/he offers to accompany her to the court room and arranges for a free legal aid lawyer for her. The social worker also contacts a specialist Domestic Violence Housing Agency to arrange for safe accommodation for this woman, where her partner will not know where she is. Once the woman has settled in, she arranges a crèche for the baby, so that she can return to work. She continues counselling with the social worker. She needs reassurance that leaving a violent partner is acceptable. She does not have to endure such abuse. If the woman is a migrant woman, the social worker will need to take her cultural background into consideration (see Chapter 7). This case is an example of where it takes a woman time to make up her mind that she cannot live with a violent man and needs to make plans for her future.

Mental health setting

A young woman of 30 is brought to the A & E Department of a large general hospital as a result of a suicide attempt. She has taken an overdose of her antidepressant tablets. She is not able to talk to the nursing, medical or social work staff, but when well enough is transferred to a mental health facility. She is then screened (using a routine abuse screening tool) and discloses that her husband controls her, does not allow her to work, controls all the money in the family, and does not allow her to visit family or friends. She has become deeply depressed as a result of this coercive control, and was given a prescription for antidepressants by her GP, who did not ask her anything about her home life as her husband came to the surgery with her. The social worker is then asked to see her. She is deeply depressed about the manner in which she has to live, but is too terrified to leave her husband, as he has always said he will kill her if she attempts to leave him. The social worker works to develop a relationship of trust with this young woman, and sees her every day she is in the hospital. Her husband visits her daily, and blames the GP for giving her antidepressants. No one confronts him as his wife is too terrified to report that she has told the staff about the abuse and threats she is experiencing. She remains in the hospital for three weeks, and then is asked to return to an empowerment group (on her own) on a weekly basis. She meets the social worker on each visit, and after three months is able to begin to review her life with her husband. She takes very careful tentative steps. She develops a safety plan (see Chapter 5) and a long-term plan. The social worker now uses narrative therapy to explore the meanings she attaches to this oppressive experience. She slowly decides to leave her husband, moving to a new location in another city where he cannot find her. She carries an emergency alarm all the time (that her husband cannot see), so that she can alert others if she is attacked by him. She very slowly and carefully makes her plans, with her social worker's help, while all the time her husband thinks she is being very submissive. Eventually she feels able to move out of the home when he is at work and moves to another city. The social worker has set up a liaison with a domestic violence agency in this city, where she is renting an apartment. She is also referred to a psychiatrist in this city to ensure she is keeping well. She finds a job she likes, and files for divorce from her husband. She completes her divorce papers 'care of her solicitor', as she does not want her husband to know where she lives. She does not attend the court case – she is still terrified of meeting her husband. She is granted a divorce and continues to live in an alternative city, with a job and new friends. She attends a women's support group, but is always careful to ensure she is not being followed, particularly at night. As the research quoted above shows, moving on from such a disempowering and learned helplessness scenario may not resolve her mental health issues, but she is better placed to live her life the way she wants.

The role of the social worker in this scenario is manifold. She needs to work at developing a trusting relationship (which means not judging this woman's experience), liaising with a range of services (legal, domestic violence, empowerment services) and encouraging this patient that she can make changes, even though they may be very slow. Without this form of intervention this woman would return to her abusive husband, remain with him, and possibly repeat her suicide attempt, or be murdered by her partner if she attempted to leave without support.

Conclusion

This chapter has explored the impacts of intimate partner violence on women's physical and mental health. It has also explored the implications for pregnant women and has outlined approaches that may be taken when working with women in this range of settings. It has outlined the guidance suggested by the WHO, which includes training all staff who may come in contact with abused women. It has suggested that screening tools are important to assess the cause of women's injuries, and highlighted the importance of keeping accurate records in case they are needed by a woman who may wish to take her partner to court. Photographs are extremely helpful for women in these situations. The chapter has also explored three possible scenarios, in three medical settings, outlining good practice, which respects the woman's decisions and her wish to leave or remain with her partner.

7   Women with special needs

This chapter will explore particular approaches for women who have special needs, such as disabled women, migrant women, members of the Travelling Community and older women. Such women may be at increased risk of abuse and will require particular interventions, alongside the range of other interventions discussed in the previous chapters. Such women have particular needs which need to be understood by all social workers and other professionals working with abused women. It is essential that social workers are aware of the complexities, which exist for all abused women, but which are particularly difficult for women with disabilities or ethnic minority women.

Disabled women

The issue of intimate partner violence against disabled women is perhaps one of the most unresearched and misunderstood areas of domestic violence (Hague *et al.*, 2011). Both women with physical and women with intellectual disabilities experience high rates of such violence. In a study in Canada (Binney *et al.*, 1988), it was found that 40% of respondents had been raped, abused or assaulted; 53% of women who had been disabled from birth or early childhood had been abused. Nosek *et al.* (2010), writing in the USA, found that women with disabilities often do not report instances of abuse for reasons including fear of retribution, feelings of shame or believing she deserved the abuse. In a study conducted by Cockram (2003) in Australia, it was found that 50% of those interviewed with disabilities experienced physical abuse and 46% experienced financial abuse. Of the women, 39% had experienced stalking, while 32% had experienced threats to their children, and 29% experienced threats to withdraw care (see Table 7.1).

They found that 43% of the abuse was perpetrated by male partners (11% by female partners). They also found that some abuse was perpetrated by family members, carers, and even 1% by clergy. These levels are clearly higher than those for the majority of women abused by intimate partners. Studies in the UK suggest that 50% of disabled women may have experienced domestic abuse during their lives (Magowan, 2004). There is also evidence that disabled women, regardless of age, sexuality, ethnicity or class, may be assaulted or raped at twice the rate for non disabled women (Sobsey and Doe, 1991; Magowan, 2004). The 2006 British

Table 7.1 Types of violence experienced by women with disabilities

Type of violence	%	Estimated number of women
Emotional: e.g. threats, harassment, constant put downs, insults	72	513
Social: e.g. controlling access to family, friends and phone calls, removing or controlling communication aids	55	395
Sexual: e.g. vaginal, oral & anal rape, being forced to take part in other sexual acts that the woman does not want to, sexual harassment	58	360
Physical: e.g. kicking, hitting, choking, cigarette burns, using weapons	50	355
Financial: e.g. no input in decisions re income, not having access to money for personal use, not allowed to have own bank account, not allowed to purchase items for children	46	325
Stalking: e.g. constantly followed, watched in a threatening manner	39	275
Threats to third parties: e.g. children	32	230
Threats to withdraw care as punishment or a means of control	29	205
Discriminatory practices: e.g. withholding or forcing medicine, removing wheelchair or battery from wheelchair, criticisms relating directly to woman's disability	27	190
Spiritual deprivation: e.g. being prevented from or forced to participate in religious or spiritual practices, being told God made a mistake	9	70

Source: www.wwda.org.au/silent7.htm

Crime Survey also suggests that having an illness or disability was associated with all types of intimate partner violence (Jansson *et al.*, 2007).

In a study by Thiary *et al.* (2012), they also set out to discover the levels of abuse experienced by disabled women in the UK. Their study was conducted between 2005 and 2008 and involved interviews with abused women and service providers. All of the women they spoke to described sometimes extreme physical abuse as well as the accompanying degradation and emotional abuse they were subjected to. As one woman described her experience: 'There was slapping on the face, chucking me out of the wheelchair. And he grabbed me around the neck' (Thiary *et al.*, 2012: 37). Their study contains a great deal of detail of the kinds of abuse women experienced (including from caregivers, not always intimate partners). As in other forms of abuse, isolating a woman from her family and friends was also a tactic used by intimate partners. In the case of abused women 'isolating a woman from other external carers was often a deliberate abuse strategy which increased women's isolation and created greater dependence, multiplying the effects of neglect' (Thiary *et al.*, 2012: 39). As one women described it: 'He was telling me who I could see. Where I could go. I mean, part of that is about being a woman, but a lot of it was I couldn't go anywhere unless he took me' (Thiary *et al.*, 2012: 41). Sexual violence was also experienced by many of the abused women, which they told no one about until these interviews. Women gave numerous accounts of constant and unrelenting forced sex and repeated rape by their partners (Thiary *et al.*, 2012: 37). It is clear from these studies that intimate partner violence against disabled women is ignored, possibly because the carer 'grooms' the health visitors or social workers involved. It is also very difficult for abused women to access services: as one disability worker in Cockram's (2003) study stated:

> There is a multiplicity of discriminations against women with disabilities. It's hard enough to access services anyway, but with restricted mobility, mental comprehension or speech impairments of some victims, it is even harder. I have had experience with many women who are extra reliant on their partners and fear having nowhere to go and no one to look after them should they leave.
>
> (Cockram, 2003: 10)

These issues were also raised by Thiary *et al.* (2012). They suggest that agencies which deal with disabled women and agencies which deal with domestic violence should liaise more and ensure that workers in both agencies are aware of the difficulties that disabled women face in leaving their homes, which may have been adapted for them, or in losing their paid carers. They suggest that good practice:

> suggests that the equality training offered needs to use both the social model of disability and gendered understandings of domestic violence and abuse, to be culturally sensitive, to be aware of issues of diversity and difference, and, if possible, to be delivered by disabled women themselves with expertise in this area.
>
> (Thiary *et al.*, 2012: 139)

As in Cockram's study, they also suggest that better services and better partnerships between the service providing sectors involved are needed. They list a series of suggestions that are essential for social workers working with disabled women:

- Be informed about disabled women's needs.
- Take advice from, and consult with, disabled women.
- Develop accessible services.
- Provide accessible well-publicised domestic violence services (including refuge accommodation) that disabled women know about.
- Do not threaten disabled women with institutionalisation if no refuge space is available.
- Develop good accessible alternative accommodation, both temporary and permanent, plus support to use it.
- Develop disability equality schemes and reviews with input from disabled women.
- Take disabled women seriously and avoid being patronising.

It is clear from these recommendations that closer links are needed between domestic violence and disability services, with better publicity about the vulnerability of disabled women to abuse. For social workers in these areas, clear understandable questions about abuse (such as an appropriate screening tool) are essential if the high rate of such abuse is to be tackled. Clearly also, more accessible refuge accommodation is essential if women are to be able to leave abusive situations. Training and awareness in both social work and disability services is essential if such levels of abuse are to be tackled and women are to be supported to live violence free lives. As Thiary *et al.* (2012) point out, a disabled women is doubly or trebly vulnerable – she is open to more frequent and additional forms of abuse, she is trapped in the abuse, the services that could help her do not exist or are not appropriate or she does not get to hear about them, other people automatically side with her abuser (as either self-sacrificing partner or a paid quasi-professional) and, if she complains, she is calling her entire care package and her independent life into question (Thiary *et al.*, 2012: 171). This is almost impossible for a disabled woman to face, which is why such women are abused and remain silent about it, fearing that that they will be institutionalised if they speak out. It is essential that social workers are aware of such vulnerability amongst the disabled community.

Intimate partner violence and ethnic minority women

Research indicates that common experiences can be identified among ethnic minority women in domestic violence situations and that responsive social work and other service provision requires an awareness of, and sensitivity to, such experiences. In reviewing this research, however, it is important to acknowledge that psychosocial, economic and cultural factors can interact in complex ways to place ethnic minority groups at increased risk of domestic violence without ethnicity necessarily being a risk factor in and of itself. It is also important to recognise that there is considerable diversity among different ethnic groups in terms of the prevalence, nature and impact of domestic violence (Allen and Forster, 2007).

Culture

Attention is drawn in the literature to the fact that there are varying cultural perceptions of what constitutes abuse (Ahmad *et al.*, 2004; Wenzel *et al.*, 2006). A point of emphasis is that cognisance must be taken of the cultural norms and values that foster violence against women, and that ethnic minority women must be able to voice their concerns about how violated they feel within a cultural framework that is meaningful to them (Asylum Aid, 2002; Sokoloff and Dupont, 2005a). Certain culturally mediated factors can be influential in deterring ethnic minority women from disclosing abuse or seeking assistance. These factors include gender roles, familism, inter-family structures, shame and collectivism. A range of studies, for example, of ethnic minority communities in the UK and USA indicate that abused women often live within a cultural milieu that makes them fail to recognise intimate violence as a social problem (Ahmad *et al.*, 2004;

Bui, 2003; Hicks, 2006). They can also face tremendous cultural pressures when they attempt to break from the cycle of abuse (Hicks, 2006). Because certain cultural traditions emphasise family privacy and require the individual to turn first to her family, seeking help in the community means confronting cultural prohibitions against causing 'loss of face' for oneself and one's family (Bui, 2003). Such studies also suggest that women do not always receive family support when they decide to leave their abusive husbands because a woman is judged to have failed in her role if she cannot maintain her marriage and provide her children with a father, regardless of his conduct (Dasgupta, 2000; Hicks, 2006). A woman's desire, therefore, to protect the family name and to avoid ostracism from her community can prevent her from seeking help outside her family.

As a consequence of these cultural perspectives, women may be reluctant to report their experiences of abuse because domestic violence is not acknowledged as a social problem within their communities or because it is traditionally viewed as a private matter. Reluctance to engage with services may, in consequence, emanate from fear of bringing shame on their families or from apprehension about sanctions or rejection by extended family networks. Secondly, the centrality of family in the lives of many ethnic minority women as well as cultural prescriptions in relation to the primacy of their roles as wives and mothers mean that, for some women, family unity pre-empts individual safety. How a woman perceives and manages her experience of domestic abuse can, therefore, be strongly influenced by culturally specific factors in particular communities.

Racism

Racist beliefs and practices can also serve to prevent minority women from seeking or finding effective interventions. Because of the experience of stereotyping and discrimination when seeking assistance, women from ethnic minority groups can feel unprotected by the domestic violence, social service, health or criminal justice systems (Bent-Goodley, 2005; Kasturirangan *et al.*, 2004). Furthermore, their experience as victims of racial prejudice by majority group members may make family and community ties all the more important (Dasgupta, 2005). In addition, institutionalised racism can operate in covert and overt ways to perpetuate exclusionary practices in services and to subtly render domestic violence in minority communities invisible (Hamby, 2005).

The notion that domestic violence is 'cultural' for some communities and, therefore, does not warrant a serious response from agencies has been documented as a significant factor placing ethnic minority women at great risk from violent partners or family members (Bograd, 1999; Burman *et al.*, 2004; Donnelly *et al.*, 2005; Sokoloff and Dupont, 2005a, 2005b). In this context, it is noted that when domestic violence is defined as culturally normative, the victimisation of women is denied, and this translates into a failure to recognise the need for intervention strategies (Dasgupta, 2005; Sokoloff and Dupont, 2005a, 2005b; Volpp, 2005). If service providers characterise ethnic minority groups as inherently violent, they tend to view intervention efforts as futile (Burman *et al.*, 2004). Stereotypes may also lead professionals to underestimate the impact of abuse on minority women or to overestimate the ability of these women to cope (Donnelly *et al.*, 2005). Furthermore, the internalisation of stereotypes may contribute to some minority women not perceiving themselves as victims of abuse or as being in need of help (Nash, 2005).

The evidence in the literature also indicates that women from ethnic minority groups typically experience anxiety and lack of trust when they engage with services because of well-founded expectations, if not actual experience, of racist attitudes and behaviour. In particular, the point is consistently made that women with a devalued racial identity feel ambivalent about using the police to deal with domestic violence because they fear that calling the police will subject their partners to racist treatment by the criminal justice system as well as confirming racist stereotypes about their own community (Bent-Goodley, 2005; Dasgupta, 2005). The literature specifically highlights the twin problems of aggressive policing and of under-policing, as well as the issue of intrusive and coercive interventions by child welfare agencies, as being key factors in deterring ethnic minority women from engaging with services (Campbell *et al.*, 1997; Pittaway, 2004). Racism, therefore, can make it appreciably more difficult for ethnic minority women to access the resources they need to escape domestic violence.

The cultural setting in which intimate partner violence occurs affects the way women experience it. For some ethnic minority women, there may be strong religious and cultural sanctions for leaving or divorcing their husbands. These issues include:

- the central role of the family in many cultures;
- the indissolubility of marriage in some religions/cultures;
- women applying for asylum status may not feel be able to (or in some jurisdictions may not be able to) apply for asylum as single or separated women;
- racism against minority cultures may inhibit women from disclosing abuse as they may fear the actions of the police or the courts.

Refugee women, if separating from their partner, may fear losing their right to stay in this country and may have been threatened with this. They may fear that their immigration status may be challenged or that they or their children will be abducted and taken abroad. These are realistic fears and should be taken seriously. In these cases, the woman should be encouraged to seek legal advice.

In both Britain and Ireland a number of specialist organisations have been established which support immigrant women experiencing abuse. In Britain, the Southall Black Sisters in London is a very well-known organisation which has been supporting African and Asian women experiencing domestic violence. Their outline of the forms of abuse women experience corresponds clearly with the research discussed above:

Forced marriage: family members, including extended family members, who use physical violence or emotional pressure to make you to marry someone, without your free and full consent;

Threats regarding 'honour': immediate and extended family members, partners and ex-partners justifying a range of abusive and violent behaviour (listed below) in the name of 'honour'. For example, using violence to prevent you from bringing dishonour or shame upon yourself or them;

Destructive criticism and verbal abuse: shouting/mocking/humiliating/accusing/name calling/verbally threatening;

Pressure tactics: sulking; threatening to withhold money, disconnect the telephone, take the car away, commit suicide, take the children away, report you to welfare agencies unless you comply with his demands regarding bringing up the children; lying to your friends and family about you; telling you that you have no choice in any decisions, demanding more dowry;

Disrespect and humiliation: persistently putting you down in front of other people; not listening or responding when you talk; interrupting your telephone calls; taking money from your purse without asking; refusing to help with childcare or housework;

Breaking trust: lying to you; withholding information from you; being jealous; having other relationships; breaking promises and shared agreements;

Isolation: monitoring or blocking your telephone calls; telling you where you can and cannot go; preventing you from contacting friends and relatives; accompanying you wherever you go;

Harassment: following you: checking up on you; opening your mail; repeatedly checking to see who has telephoned you; embarrassing you in public;

Threats: making angry gestures; using physical size to intimidate; shouting you down; destroying your possessions; breaking things; punching walls; wielding a knife or a gun;

Sexual violence: using force, threats or intimidation to make you perform sexual acts; having sex with you when you don't want to have sex; any degrading treatment-based on your sexual orientation;

Physical violence: punching; slapping; hitting; biting; pinching; kicking; pulling hair out; pushing; shoving; burning; strangling; raping;

Denial: saying the abuse doesn't happen; saying you caused the abusive behaviour; being publicly gentle and patient; crying and begging for forgiveness; saying it will never happen again;

Suicide: acting in ways which make you feel suicidal or encouraging you to contemplate or commit suicide.

This list of abuse incorporates all the issues of domestic violence listed in other sections of this work, but also includes forced marriage and honour issues.

Leaving an abusive relationship

The Southall Black Sisters also provide advice on how to leave an abusive relationship, which can be complicated by a woman's immigrant status.

If you share a home with the person who is abusing you or you are scared that they will continue to abuse you because they know where you live, for your safety and protection, you must decide whether you want to leave home for a short while or permanently or keep them out or away from your home.

In order to help you your legal adviser will need to know the following information:

- When you came to the UK and how long you are allowed to stay in the UK.

- Why you came to the UK (e.g. to join your husband, as a student, domestic worker).

- If there are any conditions or restrictions upon you staying in the UK (e.g. that you must stay married or you must not work or claim benefits.

In an emergency whether you are assisted by an organisation or the police you must make sure you collect your essential belongings, any medication you or your children take and essential documents such as passports, birth certificates and benefit books belonging to you and your children.

If you have had to leave your children behind in an emergency you should call the police immediately and ask them to escort you home so you can pick up your children safely. If they are at school, speak to the school head immediately and try and collect them. When you return home it is advisable not to get into any conversations with family members. If your children are no longer at your home, or your partner and/or his family refuse to hand the children over to you or the police are not prepared to accompany you, seek urgent advice, preferably legal advice.

They suggest that women contact the Women's Aid Federation helpline to get information on the location and telephone numbers of refuges and support services. They also provide such services for women. There are over 250 refuges across the UK. All refuges in the Women's Aid Network operate an open door policy for women and children in need. However, some refuges are able to provide services addressing the particular needs of Black and ethnic minority women. For a full list of such refuges contact Women's Aid on their 24-hour helpline. If you are an adviser you can obtain the Women's Aid Gold Book: Directory of Domestic Violence Refuge and Helpline Services from the Women's Aid Federation (Tel: 0117 944 4411).

Protection: staying at home or returning home

Staying away from home can be a very dangerous time for a woman.

You may decide that you do not want to leave home or that you only want to stay away from home until you are sure it is safe to go back.

You may be able to obtain an injunction which is a court protection order preventing your abusive partner or relative(s) from contacting you, harassing you, threatening you or harming you for a specified period. If you share a home with an abusive partner you may be able to obtain an occupation order which is a type of injunction ordering your partner to leave your home and not return for a specified period.

You can obtain emergency protection orders (injunctions) on the same or next day, if you can show that you or your children are at immediate risk of physical harm or that your abuser will prevent you from obtaining a court protection order if they know you are planning to do this.

You should get legal advice as soon as possible from a family lawyer. You will qualify for legal aid (free legal advice and assistance) if you have no income or are on benefits. If you have a low income the legal adviser will calculate whether you qualify for legal aid or you have to pay towards your legal advice costs. If your income is too high you must decide whether you can afford to pay legal advice and representation privately or if you can apply for a court protection order yourself. When seeking advice from a legal adviser you will be given an appointment and you should take proof of your income with you (i.e. benefits book, letter from benefits agency, last 3 months' payslips or a letter from anyone who is providing you with free accommodation and support).

You can also obtain advice and information from Rights of Women on 020 7252 6577 (telephone) or 020 7490 2562 (textphone) on Tues/Wed/ Thursdays from 2–4 pm and 7–9 pm, Fridays 12 to 2 pm) where free legal advice is provided by telephone by solicitors and barristers on family law issues. You can also obtain a Domestic Violence DIY Injunction hand-book in English, Bengali, Gujarati, Hindi and Urdu from Rights for Women for £6.00 which shows you how to apply for a court protection order yourself.

Sanctuary Project/Sanctuary Scheme

The Southall Black Sisters group also provides the Sanctuary Project/Sanctuary Scheme, which is a government introduced scheme that aims to make it possible for victims of domestic violence to remain in their home and feel safe.

Sanctuary Project/Sanctuary Scheme is a homelessness prevention initiative offered by a number of local authorities. They can offer you some or all of the following options to improve your safety and enable you to remain at home:

- A safety planning meeting with a specialist domestic violence adviser who can work with you to assess your needs and help you to decide whether the Sanctuary Project would help you.
- A quick and free change of locks.
- Quick (within hours) free additional home security measures such as window locks, fire-proof letter box, stronger doors.
- Adapting a room in your home so that in the event of your abuser breaking in you (and your children) can lock yourself into this 'sanctuary room' and your abuser will not be able to break into the room. You can then use a telephone or emergency alarm system to call the local police for urgent assistance. This scheme is not means tested and may be offered to you whether you live in local authority, housing association or private (owned or rented) accommodation providing you have the permission of the landlord before making any structural adaptations.

This scheme helps to support women who have experienced domestic violence and wish to remain in their homes but it should not be seen as a guarantee of safety. You need to decide whether you will be safe when you go out of your home as well as whether you will be safe whilst at home. You should seek independent advice, preferably from a lawyer, housing advice or women's advice centre if you need to discuss your safety needs.

All of this information can be obtained in the Southall Black Sisters website: http://www.southallblacksisters.org.uk/. This website also provides information on issues relating to visas and migrant women.

Ethnic minorities in Ireland

In Ireland, the equivalent organisation for migrant and African women is AkiDwA [Swahili for sisterhood]. AkiDwA is based in Dublin and takes a strong interest in issues relating to intimate partner violence. AkiDwA as an organisation emerged from regular meetings held amongst fellow migrant women, from 1999 to 2001, convened by Salome Mbugua, a Kenyan migrant woman who had arrived in Ireland in 1994. In 2001 Salome mobilised a group of African women to come together to share their experiences of living in Ireland. What emerged from this meeting were feelings of exclusion, isolation, racial abuse and discrimination, and issues related to gender-based violence were also raised. The group went on to meet regularly and were supported and offered facilitation from outside.

Like the Southall Black Sisters group in the UK, they also take an interest a range of gender-based issues. AkiDwA's gender-based violence programme focuses on female genital mutilation, domestic violence and sexual violence. They work to improve delivery of culturally appropriate support services for intimate partner violence related issues, and they provide guidance and training to migrant women experiencing domestic violence and women with medical concerns related to genital mutilation. AkiDwA advocates for legislation to prohibit female genital mutilation in Ireland, including the principle of extraterritoriality.

AkiDwA also focuses on employment issues for migrant women. They run a programme which focuses on migrant women's access to the labour market, recognition of skills, education and work experience from abroad and the impact of the current recession on migrant women and families. The attainment of economic independence is crucial for women, especially for migrant women experiencing domestic violence, so that they can make decisions-based on safety and not poverty. AkiDwA's gender-based discrimination programme advocates for the equality of treatment and engagement for migrant women through legislation, policy and practice reform and through awareness raising training and promoting balanced public debate. AkiDwA's policy work aims to progress equal access to rights, services and economic opportunities and monitors safety and protection issues, in particular within state systems, lobbying for necessary reforms. AkiDwA supports the strengthening of women's voice in civic and political structures.

Understanding gender-based violence: an African perspective

This AkiDwA research was undertaken in response to the changing client profile attending gender-based violence service providers in Ireland and to address the needs identified by women contacting AkiDwA in relation to gender-based violence issues. With regard to African women in Ireland, this survey was intended to ascertain a baseline of their understanding and perception(s) of domestic violence. Through discussions with African women, AkiDwA came to realise that this objective was influenced by the realisation that some African women only recognise the physical part of violence, such as battering, as domestic violence. In awareness raising training, AkiDwA saw in its small sample that verbal abuse and psychological/mental abuse is more or less tolerated and accepted, and not as recognised or acknowledged as a form of domestic abuse.

Domestic violence amongst migrant communities in Ireland (March 2009)

This AkiDwA survey was conducted with two target groups: African women and service providers in Ireland. The objectives of the survey were to:

- assess the women's knowledge and awareness of domestic violence;
- discover the women's experiences and views on the causes of domestic violence while in Ireland;
- identify challenges in seeking support;
- formulate recommendations on domestic violence for service providers.

The study found that the women had good knowledge of the term 'domestic violence' and an understanding of all its manifestations: physical, sexual, emotional, psychological and financial abuse. They described it as:

> any kind of abuse subjected to [a] woman by [her] husband/sexual partner within the household. This can be in form of beating, pushing one out of the door, the use of abusive language, a negative attitude such as poor communication, the woman cooking food and [the] husband does not eat and the husband coming back home late. Domestic violence can also be emotional because all women's work is not appreciated; a woman is always in the wrong.

Traditionally, the husband listens to his parents-in-law more than his wife, also causing emotional stress on the woman. Others said that 'domestic violence occurs when [the] male partner does not leave money for food, even with the knowledge that [the] woman has no source of income'. In the survey, the women also mentioned that domestic violence can be in the form of denial of rights, where they are not allowed to seek employment, and men believe that a woman should stay at home and do domestic chores. 'It is woman's job' (AkiDwA, 2008).

The causes of domestic violence while in Ireland: African women's experiences and views

Many of the women to whom AkiDwA has spoken have a history of torture and trauma. These women have the double-bind of insecure status, especially amongst refugees and women seeking asylum, and delays in obtaining legal immigration status, which only serves to increase the duration of their mental and emotional strain. The women cited the following as the main triggers of domestic violence in their experiences.

Lack of financial resources and a reduction in the standards of living is always a threat to family stability. When both partners are unemployed and are not able to work, there can be increased financial problems. The partners tend to irritate each other and get on each other's nerves. This issue is even more severe for couples in direct provision, as people seeking asylum in Ireland do not have the right to work. The husband could want to be the boss, controlling all the resources in the house, including financial resources from the woman's own paid work. The survey also revealed that some cultures fuel domestic violence within Africa. The women feared reporting incidences of domestic violence to the relevant authorities. They felt intimidated because it is African cultural tradition not to talk publicly about anything concerning domestic issues. A woman could feel stigmatised and rejected by her friends and the community if it were public knowledge that poor relations existed within her marriage. This, in turn, can lead to low self-esteem. Most women in Africa, irrespective of their marital status or educational levels, are often dependent on men to access resources such as labour, land and financial credit. They may also preserve their marital relationships for the sakes of their children and families.

When a woman does not know her rights, she will believe that everything that the man does is correct. The women in the group viewed this as self-denial. This often happens in instances where an educational difference exists between male and female partners.

Fear of alienation from family and community

It is clear that African women are not willing to seek their families', friends' or the state's support for fear of being stigmatised and alienated from their communities. Women are made to believe they cannot speak about domestic issues in public, as people who know them would contact their countries of origin, informing people back home what has happened in Ireland. It was also reported that leaving a marriage does not always appear to offer a solution for a woman within a violent relationship. Some women want the option to reconcile, which is why they prefer reporting the violence to their religious leaders in the hopes of having them inter-vene. But if the situation worsens, then the next line of action is contacting An Garda Síochána [the Irish police service].

One of the biggest issues facing African women is the issue of residency. African women whose residency in Ireland is dependent on their husbands'/ spouses' residency status face specific difficulty in accessing services on domestic violence. This may put their residency status in jeopardy, or the women may be concerned about betraying their husbands/partners, whose residency might only have temporary status. Similarly, women in the asylum process who live with their husbands/partners in accommodation centres may find it difficult to access services for fear of disclosure and how this might affect both of their applications. They may be afraid to involve the Gardai because, without the support of extended family, they worry about being left alone to support their children.

Many women reported that domestic violence services do not meet their needs. They reported racism and discriminatory responses. These kinds of experiences are likely to discourage women from seeking help. The religious leaders whom African women consult felt that their studies in theology and pastoral care were devoid of any guidance on this very sensitive issue. The religious leaders reported that they often used common sense, counselling the couple and, at times, informing them of the law. The leaders suggested that they would benefit from guidance in this area.

Many African women need mediation to address their domestic problems, and yet they go to great lengths to protect the perpetrator, to the detriment of their own safety. A barring order against a partner is often not what they feel they need, as this may lead to marital breakdown. The women feel that leaving the marriage is not a solution because they fear that their next relationship may not go well and they will end up alone (AkiDwA, 2008).

In the Dail on 13 March 2012, the Minister for Justice stated that the issue of domestic violence can be dealt with in the Irish Naturalisation and Immigration Service (INIS):

> Any person in such a situation can approach the INIS directly or through An Garda Siochana or a non-governmental organization and their case will be examined with sensitivity. All cases are addressed on an individual basis and independent status is granted where the known circumstances of the case warrant it.
>
> (KildareStreet.com, 2012)

However, while this is a welcome statement, it does not take into account the complex cultural and familial reasons which may prevent an abused woman doing this. But this is an option which AkiDwA or Women's Aid may help a woman to choose this route if she chooses to take this option.

Domestic violence toolkit

Identifying and Responding to the Needs of African and Other Migrant Women Experiencing Domestic Violence in Ireland, April 2009: this toolkit was developed in order to raise awareness and help African and other migrant women understand domestic violence and its dynamics. The toolkit was also developed to share an African cultural perspective, as well as to provide insight into the specific needs and experiences of African women experiencing (or affected by) domestic violence. It illustrates unique factors of domestic violence cases of African women living in Ireland, and highlights how better to facilitate their effective access to domestic violence support services. This is useful tool for social workers working with migrant women. The domestic violence toolkit can be downloaded from: http://www.akidwa.ie/DVToolkit2009.pdf.

Intimate partner violence in the Travelling community

In a study carried out by Allen (2012a), the experience of intimate partner violence within the Irish Travelling community was examined and explored. There is also a community of Travellers in Britain and these findings can be said to relate to them also. 'Travellers' are predominantly an indigenous European ethnic group (Cemlyn, 2008) and there are an estimated 23,681 Travellers in Ireland (Central Statistics Office, 2002). While the Irish Travelling community is not legally recognised by the state as an ethnic minority, there is a growing consensus that they are a distinct community, with traditions that differ from the majority community. As with the experience of migrant women, Travellers experience racism and are reluctant to leave their partners because of the strong 'familial' mores within the Traveller community. What is clear is that the legal and support mechanisms that have been introduced, and which are to a certain extent effective in facilitating settled women to eventually access safety from abuse, are not, for a number of reasons, as effective for Traveller women. The reasons for this lack of effectiveness lie in structural and cultural factors both within the systems themselves and within the Traveller community.

The importance of marriage, which couples tend to enter into at a young age, is underscored by the pressure exerted on both parties to remain in the marriage at whatever cost. This reflects the traditional Catholic (and other religious) family values which many older women in all communities would cite as reasons for remaining in an abusive relationship. 'If you're married, you're married to stay.'

These intra cultural pressures interact with the structural difficulties which exist in the systems and agencies on which abused women rely when seeking to access safety.

The Traveller women reported a range of help-seeking behaviours which reflect those noted in other studies (Goodman *et al.*, 2003, 2005). Many of these help-seeking activities, however, involve interaction with official systems and services which are not designed for, nor always supportive of, the nature of the Travelling community's family oriented way of life. The women believed that for the most part the Gardai/police do not want to get involved. Even if they are arrested, the women have experienced the backlash from their husbands:

> You get them arrested, and you're guaranteed the minute they get out of the police station, they're going to come back and break you up and the trailer as well. It's for shame's sake as far as they're concerned, their credibility is gone.

As recent figures show, obtaining a barring order is becoming increasingly difficult in the Irish legal system (Watson and Parsons, 2005). For Traveller women, there are added difficulties in either obtaining a barring order, or taking charges against her partner. The close-knit family lifestyle may mean that not only is a woman now confronted by an abusive husband, she may also be confronted by angry in-laws, and perhaps even by her own parents and siblings, who do not wish to see her marriage fail. She may also have literacy difficulties, which make the form filling and legal procedures necessary for obtaining a barring or protection order almost insurmountable. Added to this is the difficulty of bringing children into town, perhaps on a number of occasions, to complete this process. The delay in cases coming to court was also referred to as a barrier.

Amongst the service providers, there were a large number of responses which recognised that Traveller women experience discrimination in accessing services and networks outside the Traveller community. However, there were also a minority of comments which suggested that violence is more acceptable within the Traveller community because of 'cultural' or 'religious' reasons. For all these reasons, Traveller women experience a range of difficulties, including racism and fear, in trying to keep themselves safe from intimate partner violence. Understanding these cultural and racist issues is important for social workers working with abused Traveller women.

The following is a list of good tips for working with migrants and Traveller women.

- Violence is not inherent in minority ethnic cultures.
- For many minority ethnic groups, be it Travellers or migrant communities, their relationship with police and statutory services can be based on fear and mistrust. This puts minority women under pressure when trying to find support.
- Limited knowledge (and hence access to) the legal system creates added barriers for women.
- Inaccurate information about rights and entitlements is of advantage to perpetrators and might cause obstacles in the process of finding help.
- Seeking assistance can be especially difficult for women whose residency status is unclear. Also they do not want to endanger their partner's residency status by reporting him to the authorities.
- Language can be a significant barrier to seeking support and access to culturally appropriate and multilingual information is vital. If a language interpreter is required, employ a professional one – NOT a friend or member of the family. If only a male interpreter is available, check with the woman if this is acceptable.
- Women from minority ethnic groups often rely on their own communities (possibly including their abuser) for support.
- Support services need to work in solidarity and partnership with minority ethnic groups to remove barriers and improve services.
- Acknowledge these women as experts on the issues of violence against women as it affects their lives.
- Develop specialist expertise towards minority ethnic groups and recognise and plan for diverse needs.
- It is important to find balance between recognising a woman's right to live a life free of violence and affirming ethnic identity and different needs.

(Pavee Point and the Department of Justice,
Equality and Law Reform, 2005)

Older women

Many older women who experience domestic violence are poorly served by the systems that target domestic violence and elder abuse, respectively, and the attitudes and needs of this population are poorly served. Moreover, little has been done to develop responsive community prevention and intervention programmes for older women who experience domestic violence. According to research on older women (Beaulaurier *et al.*, 2005) powerlessness, self-blame, secrecy, protecting the family, and hopelessness were seen by respondents as a contributing factor to the reluctance of older women to seek help for domestic violence or other forms of abuse. These victimisation behaviours effectively become barriers to helpseeking. Age was a contributing factor in erecting barriers to seeking help.

Older women may have experienced violence and abuse many times longer than their younger counterparts. Respondents related that there is a kind of inertia that develops in the course of a long, abusive relationship, such that change becomes extremely difficult. Also, older women may feel additional reluctance to seek help, since this would require discussing private family matters with outsiders. Repeatedly respondents observed that people of their generation did not talk about private family issues. Particularly for those older women who already feel that they are to blame for problems in the home, breaking secrecy can only exacerbate their feelings of shame and embarrassment. Hopelessness seemed to have a strong age related component that was expressed as a feeling that it might be too late, or if things had gone on 'this long' one might just as well continue to endure the abuse.

Moreover, women in the study expressed little faith that they would receive adequate services if they did speak out. Many believed that domestic violence services were targeted toward younger women, and that an older woman would be turned away. Some even thought they might be laughed at or ridiculed. There was also the added dimension that, in some cases, women with adult children appeared to fear that revealing domestic violence or abuse might disrupt their relationship with adult children.

However, the clearest age related aspect of protecting family relates to the concern that many women expressed for the abuser. Most women in the study believed that reporting domestic violence would most likely result in arrest and removal of the spouse. For many women this was unacceptable. Many believed that their abuser was 'sick' and needed treatment rather than punishment (Beaulaurier *et al.*, 2005). In Ireland many women sought the help of their local priest if they decided to leave the abusive relationship. As marriage in the Catholic faith is for life, the priest would then speak to the abusive partner, and assure the woman that it would not happen again. She would return and the abuse would continue as before. She would then feel trapped and remain in the relationship. Such an approach would not occur today, but it helped to confine older women within an abusive relationship.

For social workers who deal with older abused women (either in a hospital setting, or a dedicated service for older people) being aware of these important facts is important in supporting a woman who has experienced or is still experiencing abuse. Physical abuse tends to diminish over time, but the emotional abuse and coercive control continues. Supporting women experiencing these forms of abuse is an essential aspect of the social work task with older women. Supporting a woman to leave the relationship (and perhaps live with a family member) would provide some solace to an older person experiencing abuse. Being aware that this can continue into older age is important, even if the physical violence has diminished. Developing a range of supports for older women who may not wish to leave the relationship is also important, and keeping in touch with such a woman is extremely important.

Conclusion

Dealing with intimate partner violence is always complex and difficult. However, when working with disabled women and women from ethnic minorities, some of these complications become more accentuated. For example, as was seen earlier in this chapter, the percentage of disabled women likely to be abused by partners is much higher than the national or even EU rates. Expecting women to leave their homes and enter institutions is not an effective outcome, and strategic and well thought out responses are necessary when working with disabled women. Similarly, with women from an ethnic minority background, the complexities for these women are equally difficult. Residency fears, cultural emphasis on marriage being for life, and few or no opportunities to earn an independent income all complicate the leaving process for such women. Similarly, for older women, religious beliefs and a fear of their partners being arrested makes it difficult for such women to obtain safety. Again, well thought out and culturally appropriate interventions are essential in ensuring that such women can find safety. Being fully aware of these complexities is essential for social workers working with these women. If one is not aware, one should talk to the relevant agencies and, if necessary, refer women to such agencies. But all social workers should be aware of these complexities, and the fears and apprehensions of disabled, ethnic minority and older women.

8   Domestic violence and child protection

Perhaps the most contentious issue in social work practice is the issue of child protection and domestic violence. This is an area which has been receiving greater attention in recent times, as there is growing awareness that there is an overlap between child abuse and domestic violence. A landmark study in Ireland in 1995 showed that 64% of women who experienced violence reported that their children had witnessed the violence (Kelleher and Associates, 1995). Children who have been exposed to family violence may have long-term physical, psychological and emotional effects. The longer family violence is experienced, the more harmful it is. Children may blame themselves for the violence or for being unable to prevent it, they may try to intervene and be injured themselves, and they may become confused by torn loyalties (Barry *et al.*, 2010). Mertin and Mohr (2002) found that witnessing abuse or experiencing the abuse has similar effects on children. UK research (National Children's Resource Centre, 2003) reveals that in 90% of domestic violence incidents, children were either present when the assault was occurring or in the next room and able to overhear the conflict. Bragg (2003) found that 80% to 90% of children in homes where domestic violence occurs can provide detailed accounts of the violence in their homes. Children who live in homes where a parent or caretaker is experiencing abuse have been called 'child witnesses'. Although parents frequently believe they are protecting their children from witnessing their abuse, children living in these homes report differently. But as the research will outline, child abuse, including sexual abuse, overlaps with domestic violence to a considerable extent. A Northern Ireland study (Devaney, 2008) expresses concern that 'children are conceived of as innocent bystanders caught up in the crossfire rather than as victims in their own right' and finds that there was a clear association between child protection registration for physical abuse and physical abuse between adult household members, with 72% crossover.

This chapter will review this overlap, and will discuss the impact of abuse on children's development, their resilience, good practice in working with abused children within a domestically violent family, and some resources that are available to support such children.

Overlap between intimate partner violence and child abuse

A number of studies have explored the overlap between families which experience domestic violence and the abuse of children within these families. The relationship between men's abuse of women and child abuse has now been well established in the literature. 'Studies specifically undertaken in child protection have demonstrated a high association between child abuse and intimate violence, showing that violence towards women may coincide with being at the greatest risk' (Holt, 2003). International research has indicated a strong correlation between instances of domestic violence and child abuse. Some research indicates that child abuse and domestic violence cases overlap in 40% to 60% of cases (Garcia-Moreno, 2002).

Walby and Allen (2004) have also pointed out that the risk of domestic violence for women is nearly doubled if there are children present in the family. It is clear from research that domestic violence is an important indicator of risk of harm to children. Much of the research suggesting links between intimate partner violence and child abuse has been carried out in the USA and Australia, while British research has confirmed these findings. The summary in Table 8.1 is not inclusive of all studies in this field, but provides a short overview of the overlap of such forms of violence.

Table 8.1 Studies of violence

Stark and Flitcraft (1988) (US study)	Of 116 children who were admitted to a hospital as a result of abuse, they found that 45% of the mothers were also being physically abused.
Bowker, Arbitell and McFerron (1988) (US study)	Of 775 women who had children with violent partners, 70% of the partners also abused the children. They concluded that 'the severity of the wife beating is predictive of the severity of child abuse'.
Goddard and Hiller (1993) (Australian study)	Of 206 children admitted to the child protection unit of a hospital, domestic violence was present in 55% of the children who had been physically abused, and in 40% of the children who had been sexually abused (82% of these were girls).
Fantuzzo and Mohr (1999) (US study)	They established that children were present in households where domestic violence was occurring at twice the rate for the general population.
Osofsky (1999) (US study)	This study concluded that children exposed to domestic violence are 15 times more likely to be physically abused and neglected than children without exposure to domestic violence.
McGee (2000) (UK study)	This research found that 71% of children witnessed physical assaults of their mother, while 10% witnessed the rape of their mother.

(Continued overleaf)

Table 8.1 Continued

Cawson (2002) (UK study)	A quarter of children (26%) said that physical violence sometimes took place between those caring for them, with 5% experiencing this frequently. 13% were emotionally abused, 7% sexually abused, 44% were neglected and 23% physically abused.
Saunders et al. (2002) (US study)	Of the children living in naval families with domestic violence, 39% reported sexual abuse, 42% physical assault, and 55% physical abuse.
Farmer and Moyers (2005) (UK study)	In a study of looked after children, it was found that over half (52%) of the children had backgrounds of domestic violence.

While the rates of abuse can vary between studies for children and their mothers, as indicated by an overall figure of 45–70%, there is agreement that domestic violence is a risk factor for physical and sexual abuse of children (Holt *et al.*, 2008).

Impacts on children

Hester *et al.* (2007: 42–43) summarise the risk to children when living in a domestically violent home:

- Domestic violence is the most common context for child abuse.
- Male domestic violence perpetrators are more likely to be abusive to children, and more extremely so.
- The more severe the domestic violence, the more severe the abuse of children in the same context.
- Children may experience multiple forms of abuse.

The evidence of research into the overlap between domestic abuse and child abuse can jeopardise the developmental progress of the children. Exposure to violence may have varied impacts at different stages of the child's development, but early and prolonged exposure can potentially create more severe problems because it affects the subsequent chain of development (Holt *et al.*, 2008). Kolbo *et al.* (1996) found in their mid-1990s review of the research literature that children who witness domestic violence are more likely to 'be at an increased risk for maladaptation' (Kolbo *et al.*, 1996: 289). A more recent US study also found that children who witnessed domestic violence had significantly worse outcomes than comparison groups who had not witnessed such violence. It was found that 62% of child witnesses were not faring as well as the average child (Kitzmann *et al.*, 2003).

Evidence has shown that pre-schoolers who witness violence have more behavioural problems (aggressive and possessive behaviour), social problems (poor social skills), post-traumatic stress symptoms (which may explain the frequency of illness in these young children), greater difficulty in developing empathy, and poorer self-esteem than children who have not had these experiences (Barry *et al.*, 2010). For infants and young children, distress may manifest itself in excessive irritability, regressed behaviour around language and toilet training (Osofsky, 1999), sleep disturbances, emotional distress and a fear of being alone (Lundy and Grossman, 2005). Lundy and Grossman (2005) analysed data from 40,636 children (aged 1–12 years) between 1990 and 1995 from 50 domestic violence agencies. They found that these young children appeared to have difficulty separating from their parents, perhaps reflecting problematic attachment issues. Martin's (2002) review of the literature also suggests that the dynamics of domestic violence can undermine the child's developmental need for safety and security, as a result of problematic attachments and their developmental needs for safety and security, resulting in difficulties getting comfort from their mothers. He also suggests that if this pattern is not interrupted, the child will be chronically overwhelmed and it may lead to the intergenerational cycle of domestic violence. For young children the impacts of domestic violence are greatly amplified as they are completely dependent on their carers for all aspects of their care. The outcomes for them can include post-traumatic stress symptoms, behavioural and social problems, greater difficult developing empathy and poor self-esteem (Huth-Bocks *et al.*, 2001). Martin (2002) also suggests that psychosomatic problems such as headaches, stomach aches and asthma, as well as insomnia, nightmares and enuresis, may also occur.

Older school-going children (approximately 6–12 years of age) will try and find reasons for the violence. They may also try and prevent the abuse from happening (Holt *et al.*, 2008). They may blame their father's use of alcohol, stress, or bad behaviour on their own or their mother's behalf, and this helps them cope with the idea that their father is bad or imperfect. If such inaccurate beliefs are not addressed, the child many be at risk of adopting anti-social behaviours themselves (Cunningham and Baker, 2004). This age group will also try and hide this secret from others, as they begin to interact more with other people (Alexander *et al.*, 2005). They also develop bullying habits, or can be at risk of being bullied themselves, as they may not be aware of the cues involved in such behaviour (Bauer *et al.*, 2006). The Bauer *et al.* (2006) US study found that children exposed to domestic violence at home are more likely to engage in generalised aggressive behaviour outside the home. School work may also be affected as children are too tired or often absent from school. However, the opposite may also occur, as school may be seen as a respite from home, and may be used as a way of not going home (Holt *et al.*, 2008).

Not being able to have friends around to the house is one of the stigmas of domestic abuse. As one of the respondents in McGee's (2000: 90) study described it:

But my friends won't come to my house. 'Mona I won't knock for you, we'll wait down the bottom of the road at about 8.00 o'clock, yeah, so you can come out'. Nobody would knock. Nobody would phone me because they didn't know if it was a good time to phone or a bad time to phone (Mona, aged 17).

Such isolation, fear and shame can isolate young people from their peers, making their lives even more restricted and more focused on the violence in the home.

As adolescents, the consequence of insecure attachment begins to take its toll. 'They may have an avoidant attachment style, and as a result, may not feel secure in intimate relationships' (Levendosky *et al.*, 2002). Levendosky *et al.* (2002) also suggest that such abusive relationships may lead to intimate violence on the part men and victimisation on the part of women in their adult relationships. However, it is estimated that approximately 30% of young boys who grow up in abusive homes become abusive themselves, while 70% do not. In fact, these 70% can become extremely supportive and protective of women and girls. Some adolescents cope by caring for their mothers and siblings, but this comes at the cost of a lost childhood and the possibility of severe emotional distress. It may also involve experimentation with drugs and other mood altering substances (Cunningham and Baker, 2004).

In summary, children may respond with a range of feelings and levels of distress or illness, including suicidal thoughts. Figure 8.1 is a list of effects that may affect children as they develop through the lifespan.

• Intense fear • Horror • Confusion • Children can become withdrawn from their non-abusing parent, usually their mother • They may suffer from post-traumatic stress disorder • Depression • Substance abuse • Temper tantrums • Severe anxiety • Low self-esteem • Blame themselves for the situation • Some of the children will have difficulties with sleeping or have nightmares • Regression to earlier developmental stage • Over achieving • Girls may marry men who are similar to their abusive fathers • Stealing or other juvenile crimes • Denial of any problem • Anger • Distress • Helplessness • Physically attack their non-abusing parent, usually their mother • Medical problems e.g. asthma, arthritis, ulcers, headaches, stomach aches • Bullying (bullying others or being bullied) • Eating disorders • Inability to concentrate • Suicidal thoughts/attempts • Children may feel ashamed • Isolation from friends • They may lose interest in school or have poor school attendance/performance • Experience multiple school problems • Side with perpetrator • Boys as adults may see it as normal behaviour to abuse their girlfriends or wives • Eating disorders • Girls at risk of early pregnancy as a possible escape from home situation (Barry *et al.*, 2010)

Figure 8.1 List of possible effects of abusive relationships on children

Double level of intentionality

In what Kelly (1996: 123) calls the 'double level of intentionality' – 'that an act directed against one individual is at the same time intended to affect others' – the intention of the abuser is that the abuse of the children will have a directly abusive impact on the woman. In Hester and Radford's (1996) study they found that children were forced to further the father's abuse. One woman described his father's pressure on his son to abuse his mother, even though he was crying and protesting that he had to do this:

> He made them kick and punch me and they did because they were so fright-ened of him. (My son) kicked me, he punched me in the face. But, when he had done it his father told him he hadn't done it hard enough, and he was to go and put his shoes on and do it harder.
>
> (Hester and Radford, 1996: 10)

Men may also threaten to kill the children if the woman threatens to leave or take them with her. In fact, domestic violence is one of the causes of the murder of children. This was clear in the case of Maria Colwell at the hands of her father in 1974. In the cases of Sukina Hammond and Toni Dales, both in the late 1980s, there was ongoing violence on the part of these men to the children's mothers (Hester *et al.*, 2007: 46). Serious case reviews in the UK have also found clear evidence that domestic violence in combination with addiction and mental health issues has been a significant factor in cases of child deaths and serious injuries to children.

Resilience

Just as women 'resist' violence in the home by their partners, children may also develop resilience against such abuse. A secure attachment to the children's mother (or another caring adult) can provide a protective resource for the child. Levendosky *et al.* (2002) found that a supportive relationship with an adult family member served as a protective factor. Relationships with peers and friends can also help to protect children from stress.

Levendosky *et al.* (2002) also found that adolescents who live in high domestic violence families are more likely to mix with violent adolescents, while those in low domestic violence households are more likely to benefit from social support. As McGee (2000) points out, school may also act as a form of social support, as children may gain high levels of self-esteem, which allow them to escape the family violence.

Summary of impacts on children

A UK study (Abrahams, 1994) highlighted a number of factors which affect the impact on children and their responses to the violence they witness:

- the frequency and severity of violence children have witnessed being inflicted on their parent, either through overhearing or through observation;
- the length of time child has been exposed to such violence;
- issues relating to race, culture, age, gender, disability, sexual orientation and socio-economic factors;
- whether the child has any outside support from extended family, friends or community;
- the nature of external interventions from agencies or community, e.g. a sympathetic teacher, while not able to prevent domestic violence, can do much to boost a child's self-esteem;
- whether children blame anyone, including themselves for the violence;
- whether children perceive violence as a way of getting their needs met;
- whether there is inconsistent punishment from the mother or father;
- whether the abusive parent manipulates family relationships;
- the quality of the mother's relationship with the child.

Indicators that children may be experiencing violence (as witness or victim) include:

- aggressive behaviour and language, precocious language – often the only indicator of violence in the home;
- anxiety, appearing nervous or withdrawn;
- difficulty adjusting to change;
- psychosomatic illness;
- restlessness;
- bedwetting and sleeping disorders;
- 'acting out', e.g. cruelty to animals;
- excessively 'good' behaviour.

(Barry *et al.*, 2010)

Social work responses to abused women

A number of recent studies and reports have highlighted the level of domestic violence within child abuse cases. Ferguson and O'Reilly's report *Keeping Children Safe* in 2001 provided evidence of the prevalence of domestic violence in child protection work. In 7% of 286 cases referred to social work teams, domestic violence was the main reason for the referral. In a further 19% of cases, domestic violence was cited as a child protection concern. This increased to 32% upon investigation.

It will be helpful to review the professional social work response to women experiencing intimate partner abuse from two perspectives. The first perspective will provide an overview of a number of relevant studies which have used either clinical/caseload samples, or case-file reviews, to explore and assess the way abused women have interacted with mainstream social work services. The second perspective will draw on reviews of social work literature to provide an insight into the professional discourses which may have influenced the practice responses and outcomes which have been found in the former studies.

In approaching the first task, two questions need to be explored: (a) do women use social work services to access support in the face of intimate partner violence?; and (b) where women do access such services, what is their assessment of this intervention? Does the literature confirm Mullender's (1996: 65) depressing contention that 'social workers have typically had a bad press as regards men abusing women', or can an alternative view be found of how social workers respond to women in violent partnerships?

Women's helpseeking

Studies which seek to delineate the patterns of women's helpseeking generally rely on evidence from studies with women in refuge services (Binney *et al.*, 1988; Dobash and Dobash, 1985; Ruddle and O'Connor, 1992), or on analysis of social workers' caseloads (Holt, 2003; Ferguson and O'Reilly, 2001). The former can be assumed to be populations experiencing severe levels of violence over a sustained period of time (Mullender, 1996: 66).

Before reviewing some of this work, however, it will be helpful to note the patterns of helpseeking reported in both Kelleher and Associates' (1995) and Watson and Parsons' (2005) Irish prevalence studies. The sources of help and support accessed by women in these studies were strikingly similar. In both studies friends and families were reported as being the most likely to be told about the abuse: 49% and 43% respectively in Watson and Parsons (2005: 76), and 50% and 37% respectively in Kelleher and Associates. Amongst formal agencies approached, general practitioners and the Gardai were the most often sought out in both studies. Interestingly, while only 6% of women in 2005 reported the abuse to someone in the Health Board, only 7% called a helpline and 4% approached a specialist support service. Kelleher and Associates reported that in their national survey only 2% approached a social worker for help (1995: 21). Their findings in the area-based study carried out with women in doctors' surgeries (as part of the national study) found a considerable difference in the figures regarding social work contact. Of the 56 women who had reported their experience of violence 24 did so to the social services, ahead of doctors, the court system, priests/ministers or refuges (Kelleher and Associates, 1995: 35). This reflects the findings of Dobash and Dobash (1985) and Bowker (1983), which show that contact with social services is likely to increase as the level of violence (and therefore injury) increases.

Refuge studies: patterns of helpseeking

Refuge studies provide more detailed analyses of the proportion of women who interact with professional social work services as a result of experiencing domestic abuse. For example, Binney *et al.* (1988: 19) found that 54% of their UK national sample of women in refuges sought help from the personal social services, while

Pahl's (1985: 80) study found that 76% had approached social workers for help, prior to going to the refuge. Dobash and Dobash's (1985: 148) larger British study found a similar figure (74%), and also found that the numbers approaching social services increased as the level of violence they were experiencing increased. Mullender (1996: 67) underscores the importance of the relationship between level of violence (and therefore danger) with the rates of social work contact. She reanalysed the Dobash and Dobash (1985) data and found 11.5% of the women made contact after the first attack, rising to 60% making contact after the most recent attack. Bowker (1983) in a study in the US city of Milwaukee also noted a rise in contacts with a range of social service type agencies as the violence levels increased. Ruddle and O'Connor's (1992) findings in the Adapt Refuge in Limerick in Ireland, suggest that 50% of the women there had contacted social workers and 25% of referrals to the refuge were made by social workers on behalf of abused women.

Caseload studies: patterns of helpseeking

The findings of studies that looked at social work caseloads display a similarly high level of contact between women experiencing abuse and social workers. In an analysis of child protection case-files in an Irish community care setting (Ferguson and O'Reilly, 2001: 30), a remarkably high figure of 55 out of 74 cases (74%) cited domestic violence as either the only problem, or one amongst other problems. Using a number of sources, McWilliams and McKiernan (1993) esti-mate that 54–75% of abused women in Northern Ireland made contact with social work services, compared with, for example, 52–80% making contact with general practitioners.

Women's assessment of social work intervention

Having made contact with social workers, what has been women's assessment of their experiences with this group of professionals? The answer to this question must be guarded, as the evidence to date is most definitely mixed. In summary, Binney *et al.* (1988), Pahl (1985), Casey (1987) and McGee (2000) report more positive experiences, while Dobash and Dobash (1985) and McWilliams and McKiernan (1993) report less reassuring outcomes. In Casey's (1987) Irish refuge sample of 127 women, 77 contacted a social worker, of whom only nine found them unhelpful. In contrast, in McWilliams and McKiernan's Northern Ireland study (1993: 66), less than one-third of the sample found contact with social workers helpful. In McGee's (2000) study of a group of 48 women (and 54 chil-dren) in Britain, 30 women made contact with social services, of whom ten were happy with the outcome, six reported a mixed result and 14 reported a negative response. What has led to these disconcerting levels of dissatisfaction with social work intervention?

The following examples give some insight into this dissatisfaction. In an Irish study by Hogan and O'Reilly (2007), they found that mothers with experience of social work involvement were extremely critical of the social work response, noting a complete absence of support. However one woman was very happy with the social work response, as the social worker met with the child, and gave the woman the support she needed. In this study they interviewed social workers who made remarks such as the following:

> As a social worker, you are well aware of the effects of long-term violence . . . That mightn't be your primary focus right now . . . Dad throws his weight around and every so often he throws mum a wallop and the kids hear this and see it. But that is not going to change right now. Right now, we need to deal with school.

Such an approach to domestic violence and its impact on the woman and children is quite shocking. Another social worker stated:

> So it's very bad – we would be saying to Mum, 'Look, your choices are very limited . . . the man has to go, or the violence has to stop. You make that decision with us or we have to step in . . . and take a much heavier hand.'

Both these responses highlight what Humphreys (2000) and others describe as 'the woman's duty to protect' the children, even though she herself is being abused and even severely beaten and controlled. Holt's study of social work interventions in domestic violence situations also highlights this emphasis on the mother's duty to protect. As one social worker emphasised: 'I think we are so narrowly focused on one issue that it prevents you from dealing effectively with anything else' (Holt, 2003: 59).

Holt (2003: 59) also refers to the pressures of the duty system. The narrow focus of the duty system was highlighted as having a negative impact on the delivery of such a service, as explained by this worker: 'Unless the person can demonstrate that it (domestic violence) was having horrific effects on their kids, they would not get an emergency response from us', while another felt resigned to the limitations of this approach to practice: 'You accept that that's the way it's going to be' (2003: 59).

Holt's findings echo a 1995 British review of child protection research (Department of Health, 1995) which also concluded that there was too great an emphasis placed on 'child protection, with too little emphasis on other avenues of family support and interventions (Department of Health, 1995: 32).

Humphreys' (2000) study of social work responses to women experiencing domestic abuse paints a very bleak picture indeed. As she states, the 'atrocity story' of severe physical abuse dominates responses to domestic violence, while the less visible forms of violence and control are ignored (Humphreys, 2000: v). In one case she quotes, a woman left her husband because of domestic violence. In a list of nine hazards for this family, the father's abuse of the woman is mentioned. The report of the Child Protection Conference failed to mention that the woman had been assaulted and the house trashed, even though this had happened only a few days before the report had been written for the Child Protection Conference. The social worker remarked:

> I can't imagine why it is not in the report . . . I can only think that I didn't think it is the type of thing that is relevant to the Children Protection Conference, particularly in making decisions about care proceedings. They are not interested in domestic violence.
>
> (Humphreys, 2000: 13)

She also refers to the Chair of a Child Protection Conference describing 'an argument between the parents', which on closer reading shows that the argument was actually a knife attack, with the woman being stabbed by her partner (Humphreys, 2000: 14).

Kelly (1996; 1994) has written persuasively about the interrelationship between woman protection and child protection, outlining guidelines for practice which avoid the exclusion of women's safety in child welfare practice. Her well-known principle that 'woman protection is frequently the most effective form of child protection' (1996: 132) is based on the well researched recognition of the overlap between the abuse of children and the abuse of their mothers (Farmer and Owen, 1995; Stark and Flitcraft, 1996; Gibbons *et al.*, 1995).

Recent research has explored the complexity of this overlap between woman abuse and child abuse, and has identified what Stanley and Humphreys (2006: 36) have described as the 'structural problem' in the delivery of services to children living with abuse and to their primary caregiver, who is usually their mother, who is also being abused. Humphreys' (2000) study of social work practice in Coventry Social Services is a good example of the challenge which this presents to good social work practice. The study utilised documentary analysis of 32 files (involving 93 children), and interviews with the social workers who had worked with the families, in order to review practice responses in the context of overlapping child and intimate partner abuse.

Her conclusions reflect much of the research reviewed previously in this chapter:

- practice was changing and varied, with examples of both good and worryingly poor practice;
- a lack of awareness by workers of the effects of domestic violence on the lives of women and children;
- a tendency to focus responsibility on the mother, while either avoiding or working ineffectively with fathers.

(Humphreys, 2000: 39)

In a 2011 study Humphreys and Absler trace the development of child protection responses over the last 130 years. They quote the work of Linda Gordon, who traced the files of charitable agencies from 1880 to 1960, and found many of the issues discussed above: 'violent men were ignored, women whose own lives were in danger were judged as inadequate when they failed to protect their children, and "child rescue" was frequently seen as the solution to protecting vulnerable children' (Humphreys and Absler, 2011: 2). Their study is based on research from 1880 to 2010 in Australia, the USA, the UK and Ireland. They come to a number of conclusions when reviewing this work:

- The invisibility or absence of the male abuser throughout the continuum of contact with the family – not being included in assessments and not being included in the intervention process – is notable.
- The invisibility or minimisation of the existence of episodes of domestic violence also becomes clear as there is no routine assessment for domestic violence; domestic violence is often referred to as 'marital conflict', an 'argument' or 'fighting'.
- If domestic violence is noted, the explanation for state inaction is that it is not part of its remit, but a private problem to be resolved by the couple. There is also the tendency to view marital breakdown as the woman's private problem which she must rectify.
- Intervention focuses on her role as mother, in relation to her responsibility for the protection of children, but not on the implications of domestic violence.
- Women are considered as primarily responsible for providing a safe environment for children and it is their responsibility to end the violence for the sake of the children. Women are given ultimatums that they leave and keep the children or stay and lose them.

Such continuous findings of mixed or poor social work responses to women experiencing abuse can best be understood by a recognition of the administrative context in which this practice is carried out. The majority of social workers in these islands work within the statutory health care and social services system, which has evolved in Ireland in a reactive manner to child abuse scandals and reports (Richardson, 2005). Official and public concerns in Ireland have led to an emphasis on child protection rather than family support or woman protection (Richardson, 2005; Buckley *et al.*, 1997). In Britain, there have been major organisational restructuring processes involving a similar emphasis on child protection, without sufficient resources to support these policy and practice priorities (Stanley and Humphreys, 2006: 38). As a result Stanley and Humphreys suggest that it is the lack of appropriate resources which is to blame for poor social worker interventions in situations of domestic violence (2006: 40).

An example, cited by Humphreys and Stanley (2006), which contains all three of the above elements was that of a long standing case from 1988, which noted the mother's drinking and neglect of the children, yet omitted to mention that she suffered such violence from her partner that she was hospitalised four times. Joint counselling with her partner was (unhelpfully) recommended at one stage, but by 1994, recognition of marital rape and assaults resulted in her being appropriately and sympathetically supported (Humphreys and Stanley, 2006: 13). According to Humphreys, the minimisation of domestic abuse through the use of language 'abounded' in the files. A knife attack and stabbing of a woman by her partner was described in one file as 'an argument between the parents'. She concludes that such avoidance of the issue of domestic violence leads to 'ineffectual' practice.

Writing in the Australian context, Breckenridge and Ralfs (2006: 113) point to the theoretical and practice split between services focusing on domestic violence and those focusing on child protection as contributing to these practice dilemmas. Just as Humphreys (2000) noted in the study reviewed above, they also point to the central focus on women as mothers, on their responsibilities to protect their children, and as the focus of blame if they cannot fully protect them from violence. In their study of 116 cases of suspected child abuse in the USA, Stark and Flitcraft (1996) found that domestic violence was the typical context for the abuse of the children, yet 'the files were silent about domestic violence'. Rather the emphasis was on 'maternal deficits' where women were held responsible when things went wrong (Stark and Flitcraft, 1996: 87). They suggest that social workers collude with this silence and that as a result abused women feel unable to disclose the abuse they are experiencing. Unable to fully protect their children from their partners' violence, but to protect themselves from the 'stigmatizing' reception they expect from social workers, women pretend that they can do so (Stark and Flitcraft, 1996: 91).

Writing on this dilemma of the 'bifurcation of practitioners' perspectives' between the rights of women and the rights of children, Waugh and Bonner (2002) found in their study of social work practitioners in statutory and non-statutory agencies that practice was underpinned by workers' theoretical understandings of domestic violence. Their comment that 'practitioners who were unclear and simplistic in their definition of domestic violence, struggled to determine who their client was and the direction of their intervention' (Waugh and Bonner, 2002: 288) identifies the fault line in professional social work interventions as assessed by the practitioners quoted in the studies cited above. They place the root of these difficulties primarily in the social workers' education, training and ongoing supervision as well as in inter-agency liaison. Stanley and Humphreys (2006) come to a similar conclusion in assessing social work practice with abused women and their children. They also identify social workers' lack of expertise in working with children and with their mothers, in order to strengthen the mother–child relationship and to reinforce the efforts women do make to protect their children, as challenges to good practice.

The Stanley *et al.* (2010) study of referrals to child protection agencies by the police found that 60% of the notified cases received no intervention, while 5% received a family support assessment or service, and 10% received a safeguarding assessment or service. The pattern which emerged was that 'families most likely to receive a service were those with whom children's services were already involved' (Stanley *et al.*, 2010: 301). Two families were referred six times, but did not receive an assessment. This again reinforces the concept that domestic violence is not seen by many social workers as the context for serious abuse.

Fear of perpetrators

In the Stanley *et al.* (2010) study, mothers were the focus in the majority of cases. Social workers were less likely to engage with fathers or male perpetrators. There was evidence of social workers talking directly to fathers/perpetrators in 63% of cases, but this interaction varied considerably: in some cases it was minimal, but in others it was extensive. As one social worker stated: 'As a general rule, I personally don't get involved with the perpetrator. Not at the time that the domestic violence has gone on'.

In general, fear of workers in confronting abusive men means that the more amenable partner (the mother) is confronted and blamed for the abuse and the risk to the children. However, such fear is not unreasonable and protective measures need to be implemented to safeguard such workers from violence and abuse themselves. As one social worker in Holt's study (2003) stated: 'I think subconsciously it's easier to deal with the woman because of the threat of violence and it's easier to dump responsibility onto her. Okay, he may not be available but I also think that it's convenient'.

The issue of grooming also needs to be borne in mind. An abused women may be so frightened of her partner that she may be unable to state what is actually happening in the home, but her partner may be very charming to the worker, making it difficult to understand that he can also be very violent. Procedures to protect social workers and others confronting abusive men need to be developed and implemented.

Good practice

A number of authors have suggested ways in which social work practice in cases of domestic violence can be improved. Holt (2003) suggests that 'Good Practice Guidelines' take the form of a booklet designed to advise social workers, in a step by step fashion. Such guidelines are being drawn up by social work staff. She also suggests using statistical information of men's abuse of women, so that clear data is available to inform the development of services. Training is also an essential aspect of good practice, and while universities are now providing such training, training on the job is also necessary to keep up to date with recent research and changes in legislation. Holt (2003) also suggests that assessment for such abuse in caseloads must be routinely carried out. This should not only involve physical abuse, but must also involve emotional abuse. A range of interagency initiatives must also be introduced to bring together different agencies working on domestic violence. The establishment of specialist posts can also keep the issue of domestic violence to the forefront of social services departments. This has been introduced in both the UK and Ireland, but with recent cutbacks (due to the international recession) many of these posts are being cut and social workers are being brought back into child protection arenas. Empowering women is another essential aspect of good practice. As one of Holt's respondents said: 'I think it's the only way of working, working on the woman, boosting her self-esteem, building up her confidence, helping her to feel it's not her fault. It's long, it's tough, it's slow, but it's very rewarding'.

Such an approach to women will make a profound difference to their ability to make reasoned decisions, which will benefit both their safety and their children's safety. Social workers must also know how to talk effectively to children so that they can disclose domestic abuse. The following guidelines are helpful when working with children.

Practice recommended for interviewing children/teenagers:

- Interview child on their own without perpetrator parent or victim parent present.
- Provide an atmosphere that supports children's comfort in discussing sensitive issues.
- Validate the children's feelings during the assessment interview.
- Provide safe and healthy coping skills and responses to domestic violence.
- Begin direct inquiry regarding domestic violence with a general statement.

Open-ended and invitational questions that can be used to explore the impact of domestic violence with children:

- How do you sleep?
- Do you ever have nightmares?
- Tell me about your nightmares.
- What is the scariest thing that has ever happened to you?
- Do you ever get so angry that you want to hurt someone?
- Tell me about what you do.

(Barry *et al.*, 2010)

Many social workers assume that if a woman leaves her partner, then both women and children will be safe. But as research shows, this can be the most dangerous time for a woman and her children. In the Stanley et *al.* (2010) study, managers highlighted the importance of longer-term involvement with such families. They quote the Jones *et al.* (2002) study which found in California a similar pattern of recycling families experiencing domestic violence through the child protective services. They suggest that domestic violence is a long-term issue, which requires long-term intervention, and highlight the need to invest greater allocation of resources to this aspect of child protection. They also suggest, as Holt and others do, that structures of assessment will need to be revisited and rethought.

Buckley *et al.* (2006b), based on their study of listening to children in the Mayo Women's Support Services, make a number of recommendations to improve services to children:

- Build a comprehensive data base of the existing services for children and young people.

- Provide direct services to children and young people who have previously or are currently experiencing domestic violence.
- An early intervention approach should be developed which should include schools, Gardai/Police services and voluntary agencies.

A module on domestic violence was introduced into the Social and Personal Education in secondary schools in Ireland. However, when a boy's father took the Department of Education to court as it did not include violence against men, the module was dropped and has not been reintroduced. Women's Aid have now introduced their 2iN2U website (http://www.2in2u.ie/), which outlines for young people the risks of coercive control in young people's relationships.

The court system also requires an overview of its work with abused young people. Most courts will give visiting rights to abusive fathers, who will continue to abuse the child's mother, either by assault when picking up or returning the child, or by sending messages to her via the children. As Buckley *et al.* (2006b) state, research into the effects of post-separation contact on child outcomes is largely quite pessimistic, as outcomes are negatively influenced by the severity of the violence exposed to. As Harne (2011: 170) points out:

> Private family law policy and practice has been one of the key areas where mothers and children have suffered because of the presumption that contact with a non-residential father is nearly always in the child's best interests. It is underlined by assumptions that violent fathers can be safe as parents and that violence against mothers ceases on separation.

The UK legislation (2002 and 2006 Children and Adoption Acts) have brought about some improvements, but Harne goes on to suggest that a change in policy to a legal presumption against violent fathers having contact or residence with their children would be a great improvement in safeguarding children. Such approaches by the Court Services in both Ireland and the UK need serious review and the voice of the child needs to be heard independently in a confidential setting.

The new revised Irish child protection guidelines, *Children First: National Guidance for the Protection and Welfare of Children* (2011), take domestic violence and the need to hear the voice of the child into account. Under Emotional Abuse and Neglect, it states that 'Exposure to domestic violence' is a form of abuse. Under Physical Abuse, it states that 'Observing violence' is a form of abuse. In Section 2.10.6 it states that 'Exposure to domestic violence is detrimental to children's physical, emotional and psychological well-being. The adverse effects of domestic violence have been well established'.

It goes on to state that:

> Children have a right to be heard, listened to and taken seriously. Taking account of their age and understanding, they should be consulted and involved

in all matters and decisions that may affect their lives. Where there are concerns about a child's welfare, there should be opportunities provided for their views to be heard independently of their parents/carers (2011: 4).

This reinforces the good practice found in Hogan and O'Reilly's (2007) study which found that speaking to the child on her own was an essential part of good social work practice. It also emphasises the importance of interagency cooperation, stating that:

> 4.1.1 No one professional has all the skills, knowledge or resources necessary to comprehensively meet all the requirements of an individual case. It is essential, therefore, that all professionals and organisations involved with a child and his or her parents/carers deliver a coordinated response. This chapter identifies the roles and responsibilities of Central Government, the Health Service Executive (HSE), An Garda Síochána [the Irish police force] and other organisations working with children. It also outlines the benefits of effective interagency cooperation.

> 5.6.3 Family support services, by way of a family support plan, may be delivered formally through the direct services of statutory and voluntary organisations, and informally through the support of extended families, friends, neighbourhoods, communities, parishes and other local networks. Where support is being provided to a family where there are child welfare concerns, it needs to be coordinated and monitored by the HSE.

Such approaches are hopeful signs that the importance of interpersonal violence in child welfare settings may become more recognised and understood, leading to better practice and better outcomes for abused women and children.

Group work

A number of agencies now provide group work for children exposed to domestic violence. This is also a hopeful and encouraging approach to tackling the longer-term impacts of such abuse and its impact on children and young people. Research has found that children and young people want opportunities to talk about domestic violence and want their accounts to be taken seriously (McGee, 2000; Mullender *et al.*, 2002). An Irish study found that in terms of investing in early interventions, violence prevention programmes targeted at children or those who influence them during early development show greater promise than those that target adults. Such early interventions have the potential to shape the attitudes, knowledge and behaviour of children while they are more open to positive influences, and to affect their lifelong behaviours.

Chris Burke from Australia uses puppets to raise awareness of the nature of domestic violence and its links with emotional abuse, physical abuse and the neglect of children. This also has the aim of changing attitudes and behaviours and promoting alternative parenting practices which nurture and support emotional and physical well being of children. This work can be found on: www. gracieproductions.com.au.

Conclusion

This chapter has examined the impacts that domestic violence has on infants, school-going children and teenagers. It has explored the difficult task of working with families in which such abuse exists, and the tendency of social workers to ignore the violence and blame women for the abuse of children. Such approaches are being increasingly questioned, but cutbacks are making it difficult for workers to provide the time that is needed to work in depth with abused women and their children. However, group work with both women and children can be a very helpful way to work with a number of clients, and raises awareness of the impact of such abuse on children. It also allows children to express their distress and sadness at the violence they have experienced or are still experiencing. Inter-agency work is essential if women and their children are to receive the long-term services they need to overcome such abuse. Liaising with agencies such as Women's Aid and refuges are essential if social workers are to provide the best service to abused children and their mothers. Domestic violence, as the research has shown, is the most common context for child abuse, and this needs to be taken into account when working with children. Assessments in child protection settings are essential if such abuse is to be identified and long-term interventions, including interagency work, are the only viable alternative to either ignoring the abuse or punishing women who are themselves being abused.

9   Perpetrator programmes

Perpetrator programmes are an area within the domestic violence services where there are some disparities of approach. There are different approaches to working with abusive men and these will be reviewed in this chapter. There is some research which suggests that mandated programmes work better than non-mandated programmes. However, one of the most important issues in working with abusive men is that couple counselling is a very dangerous approach to take. The reason for this is that a woman who is being abused is not free to say what has actually happened to her, and she will be afraid that if she does disclose what is happening at home, she will be likely to receive further assaults when they return home together. For these reasons, couple counselling is strongly discouraged when working with abusive partners. It is likely to lead the woman into greater danger and will not resolve the issues involved in intimate partner violence. Group work is seen as the best approach to working with abusive men, and one of the first and most well known of these programmes was the Duluth Model set up by Ellen Pence in Duluth, Minnesota in 1981.

Duluth Model

The Duluth Model of Power and Control, which is the basis of abusive relation-ships, was shown in Chapter 1. She also developed the Equality Wheel, which is the opposite of the Power and Control Wheel, and which is the basis of egalitarian relationships (see Figure 9.1). As Pence and Paymar (1993) point out in their overview of the Duluth Model, long-term change and a real commitment to egali-tarian relationship takes time and requires a long and honest look at deeply held beliefs. One of the strengths of the Duluth Model is that all agencies are involved in this approach, including the police, the courts, the probation service, refuges and the programme itself. All these agencies agreed that their aim was to confront and eliminate violence and not act as abuser advocates. The programme lasts for 26 weeks, and most of the men attending are court mandated. Only 10% of those who are not mandated by the court complete the programme. There is an intake process where the man's level of violence is assessed, his history of drug or alcohol use, his likelihood to disrupt the group, his use of violence towards his children and his understanding of his contract (that he will sign), and the release of information from one agency to another. As Ellen Pence states in Miller (2001), the programme is based on literacy approaches of Paulo Freire. They also use short video vignettes, and the purpose of these 'is to make a connection between these video scenarios and their own abusive behaviours' (Miller, 2001: 1009).

The objectives of the Duluth Curriculum are as follows:

- to assist the participant to understand that his acts of violence are a means of controlling his partner's action, thoughts, and feelings by examining the intent of his acts of abuse and the belief system from which he operates;
- to increase the participant's understanding of the causes of his violence by examining the cultural and social contexts in which he uses violence against his partner;
- to increase the participant's willingness to change his actions by examining the negative effects of his behaviour on his relationship, his partner, his children, his friends and himself;
- to encourage the participant to become accountable to those he has hurt through his use of violence, by helping him acknowledge his abuse, accept responsibility for its impact on his partners and others, and take specific steps to change;
- to provide the participant with practical information on how to change abusive behaviour by exploring non-controlling and non-violent ways of relating to women.

(Pence and Paymar, 1993: 30)

Each week different aspects of the issues raised on the Power and Control Wheel are raised and examined. There are eight themes on the Equality Wheel and these are discussed over a three-week period. There is also a women's support group in which women can also discuss the abuse and control they have experienced. The Power and Control Wheel was developed by the Women's Group, because they are best at understanding what abusive relationships are and how they affect women:

> Women said these are the things they want men to talk about, the ways they are treating them – how they use intimidation, how they isolate, how they use money, and how they use the children. They want them to talk about sexual abuse and physical abuse.

(Miller, 2001: 1009)

The group also keep a log of their actions towards their partners. As Pence says:

> In the first part of the log, we try to broaden the men's ideas of what abuse is. Then we try to help the men understand what makes something abusive and the context in which behaviours occur that make them intimidating or coercive or abusive.

(Miller, 2001: 1014)

As Gondolf (2012) points out the Duluth programme is based on a gender-based orientation and cognitive behavioural approach.

The recent Duluth website outlines the advantages of using the Duluth Model.

A community using the Duluth Model approach:

- has taken the blame off the victim and placed the accountability for abuse on the offender;
- has shared policies and procedures for holding offenders accountable and keeping victims safe across all agencies in the criminal and civil justice systems from 911 to the courts;
- prioritizes the voices and experiences of women who experience battering in the creation of those policies and procedures;
- believes that battering is a pattern of actions used to intentionally control or dominate an intimate partner and actively works to change societal conditions that support men's use of tactics of power and control over women;
- offers change opportunities for offenders through court-ordered educational groups for batterers;
- has ongoing discussions between criminal and civil justice agencies, community members and victims to close gaps and improve the community's response to battering.

(http://www.theduluthmodel.org/about/index.html)

Other models of programmes

The Duluth Model has been the model for perpetrator programmes in many countries. However, not all programmes are run on this model. As Wood *et al.* (2010) and Gondolf (2012) point out, other programmes use anger management, psychodynamic counselling, stages of change or motivational counselling or even couple counselling. They also suggest that as there is a strong correlation between alcohol and drug use and severe intimate partner violence perpetration, some programmes may address substance misuse individually. Wood *et al.* (2010) report that international evaluations of this type of approach have been positive. The most common of these approaches are social learning and profeminist approaches which were found to be the most common modalities for batterer programmes (Shamai and Buchbinder, 2010). As they point out, there are two main approaches to such programmes: (a) programmes that emphasise the acquisition of new attitudes toward violence and the misuse of men's power over women, to alter cognitions, emotions and behaviours in conflict situations; and (b) programmes that pay more attention to cognitive–behavioural aspects, focusing on issues such as anger management, including monitoring negative internal interpretations of dialogue in conflict situations, identifying signs that precede a violent episode and techniques for controlling violence (Shamai and Buchbinder, 2010: 1339). Group work is helpful because it provides a framework for meeting other men struggling with similar problems. This reduces men's social isolation and encourages self-disclosure (Edelson and Tolman, 1992).

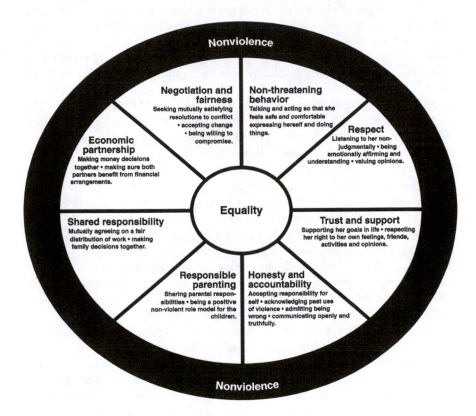

Figure 9.1 The Duluth Equality Model.

International research

Shamai and Buchbinder (2010) conducted a study in Israel of a number of batterer programmes, which seem to be based more on cognitive behavioural approaches, and which were all run by qualified social workers. Each group included from 7 to 12 participants, both voluntary and mandated by the courts. In their findings three themes seemed to emerge from the research: (a) therapy as a learning context, with the therapist as teacher and father and the group as a context in which learning takes place; (b) therapy as a source for learning self-control; and (c) therapy as turning point (Shamai and Buchbinder, 2010: 1344).

They found that for the most part the therapists were seen as 'placing them above the men' (Shamai and Buchbinder, 2010: 1345). They were for the most part looked up to and revered. Most of the men disassociated themselves from the group to begin with. They used a 'dividing or splitting strategy to disengage from the aggressive parts in himself, and looked on the other members as representing evil' (Shamai and Buchbinder, 2010: 1346). However, those who overcame these fears experienced the group as a safe place that enabled learning. However, the primary learning that took place was 'a time out' approach, which many of the men thought was a very good means of controlling their tempers and violent behaviours. They continued to blame their partners for causing the problems at home, taking no responsibility on themselves. As Shamai and Buchbinder point out: 'although the men regard the acquisition of self-control as the growing success of the treatment, the power-based schema is present in their references to it' (2010: 1349). While self-control is seen as a plus from the programmes, the coercive control which underpins intimate partner violence is still there. As the authors suggest, the men mentioned their wives as responsible for their violent behaviour. 'The power posture adopted towards wives before therapy was not transformed (Shamai and Buchbinder, 2010: 1352). As the authors also say, the men were not aware of their inner beliefs regarding power in human relationships in general and intimate gender relationships in particular (Shamai and Buchbinder, 2010: 1354). This raises the question of to what extent the patriarchal beliefs of these abusive men are challenged in these groups and to what extent 'time out' can actually last if their belief systems do not change. 'But the findings do not indicate a profound change in the basic scheme of interpersonal relationships' (Shamai and Buchbinder, 2010: 1356). Wood *et al.* (2010) also suggest that as there is a strong correlation between alcohol and drug use and severe intimate partner violence perpetration and some programmes may address substance misuse individually. They report that internationally evaluations of this type of approach have been positive.

Gondolf addresses many of these issues in his new book *The Future of Batter Programmes: Reassessing Evidence-based Practice* (2012). He addresses the issue of the use of psychodynamic programmes, change stages and motivational interviewing and suggests that the modern approach to many of these programmes is that 'batterer programmes don't work' (Gondolf, 2012: 46). Having reviewed much of the research into these approaches, he comes to the conclusion that 'there is yet no gold standard evidence that any of them are more effective overall with batterers than current programmes' (Gondolf, 2012: 48). He also suggests that that batterer programmes should be more closely linked with the courts, the rest of the criminal justice system and other community services.

Perpetrator programmes in Britain

As Mullender (1999) has pointed out, within Britain, those most likely to provide projects for abusive men are the probation service and voluntary bodies. This is also the case in Ireland, where a number of voluntary organisations and some probation services provide such projects. Some organisations in Britain only accept court mandated clients, while other can be self-referred, or use a combination of mandated and self-referred clients. As Mullender (1999: 225) states:

> the key issue in seeking a satisfactory groupwork model for abusers is the extent to which they must work with men's denial and minimisation of what they have done. There is a grave danger in adopting any approach that is not

sufficiently confrontative in style and feminist in orientation to cope with the fact that much of what abusive men contribute in groups – until they are heavily challenged by the workers and by one another – is a gross distortion of reality.

This is an important point, as abusive men will blame their partners for their behaviours. In a study by Hearn (1994), he found that men could be extremely violent, (including threats of rape, torture and murder), but they all suggested that they had positive attitudes to women. Denial involves forgetting, blanking out and excluding particular forms of abuse as not of any importance. In this study he found that 'confessions' often lack remorse and merge into denial, sometimes blaming the woman for falling down the stairs. As Hearn points out, the challenge for abusers groups is to ensure that abusive men not only talk about their violence, but take responsibility for it. As he states, this is the real challenge to those running abusers groups, that men take responsibility and are not learning a new language to stay in control.

As Straus (1979, cited in Pence and Shepard, 1988) outlines, there are three main approaches to working with abusive men: the intraindividual, the socio-psychological and socio-cultural. Gondolf (1985, cited in Nosko and Wallace, 1988: 34) listed them as psychoanalytical, social learning and socio-political. These approaches are remarkably similar. The intraindividual model has been criticised as it can lead to men justifying their behaviour. As Wood and Middleman (1992) suggest, this approach is flawed as men can control themselves by not hitting their employers, but still go home and hit their partners. As Mullender (1999: 230) states, 'An overall objection to the concept of anger management is that it feeds into men's habitual denial and minimization of their behaviour . . . it avoids focusing on the power and control inherent in the gendered dynamic of abuse'. Mullender goes on to state that most groups which use a profeminist approach also use behaviourism but with a strong cognitive overlay, regarding people as aware of what they are doing and able to make changes. The intrapsychic model sees men's abuse of women as rooted in earlier developmental problems which are compounded by past or current stress, and takes the view that these problems need to be tackled before the violence can diminish. It takes no account of the abuse women experience, and the ongoing abuse that may continue as men experience lengthy treatment. 'This is why feminist-inspired groups avoid any discussion of families of origin, i.e. past excuses for current responsibility' (Mullender, 1999: 231). Mullender goes on to outline that profeminism is not a groupwork model in itself but it is a set of beliefs that gives priority to a feminist understanding and feminist concerns (Mullender, 1999: 232). This is the approach outlined above in Pence and Paymar's (1993) Duluth Model. As Mullender (1999: 233) states, 'violence does not stem from anger but from a belief system wherein men are convinced they have to dominate and control'. These attitudes come from a long history of patriarchal oppression. Profeminism is therefore an essential aspect of abusers groups. This involves including abused partners in the work of these groups, otherwise it is impossible to access what has been happening and whether men are in complete denial, minimising their behaviour and even lying to their group leaders.

Tackling abusive fathering

Harne (2011) carried out a study into perpetrator programmes examining whether these groups tackle the issue of violent fathering. She examined four programmes: two were run by the Probation Service in Britain, and two were run by voluntary groups. Most of the members in the Probation Service groups were court mandated to attend. All of these programmes used a similar methodology, using a cognitive behavioural approach with the addition of a gender analysis 'addressing perpetrators' assumptions of dominance over women and attitudes of entitlements' (Harne, 2011: 154). The purpose of the cognitive behavioural approach was to broaden the participants' understanding of what constitutes violence and to develop empathy for their partners' perspectives. One of the voluntary programmes also included a lengthy period of psychodynamic counselling over an 8–12 week period. The justification for this approach was to enable the men 'to connect with their underlying feelings and emotions' (Harne, 2011: 154). The programmes also varied in length from 20 weeks to 56 weeks. One of the probation programmes lasted only 10 weeks but this was in the process of being extended to 20 weeks. Neither of the probation programmes sought feedback from the men's partners, but the voluntary groups did. (As will be seen such feedback is essential in ascertaining the true extent of change within such groups.) There were also other differences in approaching children's needs. One of the voluntary groups felt that fathers' motivation for making contact with their children could be dangerous, but the second group (the programme that provided psychodynamic counselling) felt that there was an 'assumption of optimism that they would be prepared to prioritize their children's needs' (Harne, 2011: 156). The probation programmes, on the other hand, did not carry out formal risk assessments in relation to child contact, but did do court reports if requested. All four programmes did some group work in relation to parenting, but this varied from group to group. As Harne states:

> these programmes therefore presented a mixed picture of practices in relation to children's safety where violent fathers were concerned. There were differences in priorities in relation to children's safety in the child contact context and how far the programmes understood the impact of fathers' violence in relation to children's fears and fathers' unwillingness to separate their own needs from those of children (2011: 158).

It was also worrying (given the range of research evidence in this context) that only one of the voluntary groups recognised the connections between a violent father's domestic violence and the sexual abuse of children.

Change?

Do men change within these four groups? One of the men who had been on the programme for 32 weeks did not understand why he was on it. He felt all he had done was love and support his family! Such lack of understanding of violence is worrying. Another man talked about having a 'a controlling problem', but went on to justify this because his partner was not doing enough childcare and housework! Some of the fathers recognised that their behaviour towards their children was intimidatory, but felt that their own views were always right. Another father stated that the work they did in the group helped him to see perpetrators as victims who need help, and could think of no circumstances where fathers should not have contact with their children. As Harne (2011: 162) notes, 'these responses raised questions about whether programmes were having any impact on these fathers in terms of changing their attitudes and behaviour'. Harne goes on to conclude that these programmes raise questions about these programmes' content about abusive parenting, and that the views of children should be taken into account if abusive fathers wish to have contact.

Women's Aid (Ireland)

In a recent report published by Women's Aid Ireland (Women's Aid, 2011) they report that in 66 calls to their freephone helpline, women disclosed that children were being abused during access arrangements. In a further 227 calls, mothers disclosed that they themselves had been directly abused during access visits. Such forms of abuse included:

- calls to tell her that her children will be killed or will never be coming home again;
- calls to say that the children have been left unattended somewhere and she should pick them up;
- calls from schools to say children have not been collected as arranged;
- children returning from access visits sad and withdrawn and saying that they do not want to go in future;
- calling late to collect children, or not calling at all on planned access days;
- returning children early or late from access.

Unfortunately, within the Irish context, if a woman prevents her children from participating in these access visits she can be jailed. Many abusive men use this as a means of further abusing the women. The courts do not listen to children's voices on whether they wish to continue access, and there is a bias in the Irish courts towards always granting access no matter how severely abused the partner may have been. These findings support Harne's (2011) study outlined above and suggest that the courts need to take a different approach to deciding on access arrangements.

Irish perpetrator programmes

In 1997, the Office of the Tanaiste published the *Report of the Task Force on Violence Against Women*. They set out core principles for the running of perpe-trator programmes:

- Protocols regarding referrals should be developed.
- Assessment procedures should be established.
- Intervention programmes should be linked to the judicial process where possible.
- There should be contact with the partner to verify the safety and well-being of the abused women and children.
- There should be limited confidentiality to allow for the sharing of any information that can advance the safety and protection of women with the appropriate persons/agencies.
- Work with men should not be done in isolation, but in full collaboration with the statutory services and women's organisations.

The authors also made recommendations for the development of intervention programmes:

- The safety of women and children should be paramount considerations in developing programmes.
- Intervention programmes for offenders should be adequately resourced and should be available in areas where support services for women and children are already in place.
- Funding intervention programmes should be based on local need and priorities.
- Contact with the judicial system should be used as a gateway to intervention programmes. Judges should have options to refer offenders for assessment, but never as an alternative to criminal sanctions nor should they have implications for the granting or duration of a barring/safety order.
- Judges in civil cases should be made aware of what programmes are available and should be able to refer men for assessment to a programme as a mandatory part of the court order.
- Existing programmes should be evaluated so that their effectiveness can be established.
- There should be a co-ordinated approach between programmes, the Courts, the Gardai and agencies providing support for women.
- Specialist training should be introduced for people to run intervention programmes.

Many of the Irish programmes were based on MOVE (Men Overcoming Violent Emotions), which was initiated in Britain.

Evaluation

In 2004, Debonnaire *et al.* carried out a review of Irish perpetrator programmes. They found that 11 organisations were running programmes and another four were preparing to do so. They also found that in one week there were 51 men in programmes around the country. The great majority of the men were not mandated by courts (see below for a discussion on this issue). They found that for most women, the emotional abuse and controlling behaviour continued after the programmes started. They also found that most men did not take responsibility for their behaviour and that although there was a decrease in violence the longer the men remained on the programme, there were men on programmes for longer than a year who were still physically abusing their partners, and the facilitators of the programme did not know about this. They found that some facilitators did not have a good understanding of domestic abuse. There was also little systemic assessment at the intake of the abusive men and it was not ongoing. There were varying levels of partner contact and varying levels of contact with women's groups. There was little involvement of the justice system, and there were not sufficient skills for risk assessment. It is clear from this evaluation that many of the recommendations made by the Task Force regarding the development of perpetrator programmes have not been met. However, as a result of this review all of the Irish programmes are now trying to follow the Respect Guidelines. (See the final section below for a discussion on this issue.)

Are court mandated programmes better than voluntary programmes?

In two important studies the issue of effectiveness of perpetrator programmes has been investigated. The question asked was whether court mandated programmes have better outcomes than non-court mandated programmes. Dobash *et al.* (2000) compared men who were sentenced to perpetrator programmes as a condition of probation with men receiving another form of sanction from the courts. The programme they examined lasted 26 weeks. After one year those who were mandated to attend the programmes decreased their physical abuse by 33%, while those sentenced to other sanctions reduced their physical abuse by only 70%. The decrease in controlling behaviour was 18% for the men on the programme, while those not on a programme deceased their controlling behaviour by 10%. Dobash *et al.* (2000) concluded from this study that there was an overall decrease in both physical abuse and controlling behaviour and an improvement in women's quality of life. In a study by Gondolf two years later (2002) he examined four different programmes, over a four year period. Most of the men on the programmes (80%) were court mandated. He explored primarily physical re-assault but also explored information on controlling behaviour and women's quality of life. He asked the question: Do men change, and if so, is this due to the programme? Gondolf (2002) found that the majority of men do stop the violence, apparently for long periods of time. These findings are based on the percentage of men re-assaulting within the last year and this decreases sharply after the first year. He found that three-quarters of the men who re-assaulted did so in the first year. At a 48 month follow-up, 90% of the men had not re-assaulted their partners for at least a year. However, at this 48 month follow-up 48% of women had been re-assaulted (cumulative approach). Interestingly, re-assault was more likely to occur while the men were still on the programme. While the majority of women reported a better quality of life, a minority were worse off. This shows that there is a group of highly dangerous men who continue to re-assault and are responsible for the most harm to women. He concludes that there is a consistent and moderate programme effect, but it is hard to quantify.

In a study by Jones *et al.* (2004), they examined three different sites and three types of programmes, which included 633 batterers and their partners (including former partners). They found that for men mandated by the courts to attend a batterers programme, completion of the programme is likely to lead to reduced re-assault. There was a 33% difference in the probability of re-assault between programme completers relative to drop outs. They also found that voluntarily enrolled men have higher rates of re-assault than the court ordered men, regardless of completion status. They found that men court mandated to attend a batterers' programme are likely to have a 50% reduction in the likelihood of re-assault. They conclude that more should be done to coerce men to attend and complete batterer programmes. 'The criminal justice system, in collaboration with batterer programmes, could more systemically monitor and respond to men's non-compliance' (Jones *et al.*, 2004: 1017).

These studies suggest that court mandated programmes have a better completion rate and are more likely to result in the reduction of re-assault. It is therefore important that more programmes adopt this court mandated approach as the outcome is clearly better – it is in fact the system that matters.

Irish study

In an Irish study (Farry, 2012) of a probation-run batterers programme, the researcher examined the responses of the men who participated and the support staff who supported their abused partners. This study examined three programmes from 2007 to 2011. Of the men who participated on these programmes, five were Health Service Executive referrals (because of child protection concerns), two were on probation for non-domestic violence (but disclosed domestic violence offences on assessment), and 17 were court mandated because of domestic violence offences. All of the men are assessed before being offered a place on the programme, and they are also given five hours of individual pre-programme work. Of the 16 men who agree to participate in the study, the average age of the participants was 35 years. One had no children, three had no contact with their children, and 12 had regular access to their children. Slapping a woman on the face, body, arms or legs was admitted to by 100% of the men; 100% also admitted to shouting or screaming at a woman; 75% admitted to having restrained a woman from moving or leaving the house; 50% admitted to kicking a woman on the body, arms or legs; 69% admitted to having threated to kill the woman; and 59% threatened to kill himself.

The feedback from the women's support workers was also very supportive of the programme. As one worker stated:

> I feel the programme has surpassed my expectations. The programme has changed so many lives of the women and children involved. The who women

were daily and sometimes hourly being harassed now have peace in their lives. They are no longer scared; their children are able to enjoy time with their fathers. The women have their friendships with the men back; they are able to build trust again. The women who are separated are using the court system for pursuing maintenance etc. without fear. The previous situations of the women have been heard and acknowledged by the programme.

Another support worker stated:

(1) A woman being able to sleep without fear of him breaking in. (2) A woman being able to talk to her partner without fear of assault. (3) The man showing the woman how to control volatile situations by his example of withdrawing from the conflict. (4) A woman going through the Court Process and completing it where she would have backed out several times previously through fear . . . All women learning that it was not their fault that they were beaten.

The aspects of this programme which seem to have helped to bring about such good outcomes are the clear referral and assessment procedures – the programme has begun to use the SARA formal risk assessment instrument specifically designed for domestic violence perpetrators – and the continued support of the District Court Judge. His continued support is vital to the success of the programme. The programme also views the safety of women and children as the paramount consideration when working with perpetrators. Taking only court mandated men or those engaged with the Statutory Child Protection Service provided that sanctions are enforced if men fail to participate. This study supports the international evidence quoted above that court mandated programmes work best with abusive partners. This programme also follows the Respect guidelines which will be discussed in the final section.

Assessment tools

Gondolf (2012) discusses the issue of assessment tools. There is a range of such assessment instruments: The Danger Assessment Scale (DA), the Domestic Violence Screening Inventory (DVSI), The Ontario Domestic Assault Risk Assessment (ODARA) and the Spouse Abuse Risk Assessment (SARA). The basic problem with many of these risk assessments is, as Gondolf suggests, the 'dynamic nature of risk' (2012: 172). Violence is more of a process than a discrete event. The best source of information is the batterer's partner, but she has most to lose by disclosing this abuse. Research has shown that structured ratings and actuarial instruments are better than unstructured or general impressions. However, the accuracy of prediction is still quite weak overall, and needs to be applied with great caution. The women's perceptions by themselves are usually better than actuarial instruments but, as we have seen above, this can place the women at a greater risk of violence and assault. Risk assessment is not a one-off, but must be updated regularly to assess ongoing beliefs and assaults. Gondolf concludes that a gender-based cognitive behavioural approach, risk assessment and supplemental treatments (for very violent men with mental health problems or those drinking excessively), court linkages that promote consistent oversight and sanctions for non-compliance, and serious efforts towards a community-based response are essential (2012: 241).

Respect

Respect is a British organisation which supplies standards, accreditation, training and research into batterer programmes. Many Irish programmes are also allied to Respect and aim to follow through their clear guidelines into making such programmes work well. Respect has a website (www.respect.uk.net) which provides clear guidelines on what works well for batterer programmes. According to their website their aims and goals are as follows:

> Respect is the UK membership association for domestic violence perpetrator programmes and associated support services. Our key focus is on increasing the safety and wellbeing of victims by promoting, supporting, delivering and developing effective interventions with perpetrators. Our services include: support, resources and training for members; managing accreditation of perpetrator programmes; developing work with young people; promoting knowledge of research about domestic violence and collaboration between researchers, practitioners and policy makers; influencing public policy; providing a national voice on masculinity and violence against women; running the Respect Phone line, and advice and referral line for perpetrators; running the Men's Advice Line, a helpline for male victims and running Dadspace.com, a virtual child contact centre.
>
> (www.respect.uk.net)

They set out the key findings from international research which guides their work.
  They have a list of guidelines which have proven to work well with abusive men's programmes:

1 Most men who take part in a well established programme situated in a coordinated community response to domestic violence stop using violence.
2 Women whose partners and ex-partners take part in programmes feel much safer and attribute this to the programme.
3 Taking part in a perpetrator programme makes criminal sanctions more effective. (They use Dobash *et al.* (2000) to support this contention.)
4 Men find the use of experiential learning helpful for making changes sustained changes.
5 Perpetrator programmes, through proactive contact with partners and ex-partners of programme participants, often make contact with and provide support to victims who do not otherwise contact or receive support from any other organisation.

6   There are several forms of mandate which help to keep them participating in programmes. Burton *et al.* (2000) support this view. They studied 351 men referred to a community-based programme in London and 76 women, who included the men's partners and ex-partners, during a two year period. As in the Irish study cited above, most of the men stopped using violence and were no longer violent after the programme, according to the women. The men found the use of experiential learning very useful for examining the effects of their violence and the alternatives to it. They also found that 'voluntary' attendance on a programme was flawed: most men were socially mandated in some way, with a perception of undesirable consequences if they did not attend, including separation from partner, social services action to remove the children or lack of contact with the children post separation.

7   Social services are now effectively operating a mandate for programme attendance, which brings more women into contact with people who can help them and provides men with ways of making changes. They use Rajagopalan *et al.* (2008) to support this. This team studied the effects of social services on 76 men mandated to participate in a community-based programme in East London. They found that almost all women engaged with the service and were provided with significant support, advice, advocacy and group support for themselves as well as providing information for case management jointly with the men's workers. Those men who participated in the programme stopped using violence, according to evidence provided by their partners/ex-partners, and most women felt safer as a result of the intervention.

8   More research is needed on the ways in which men can be most effectively assisted to stop using violence and other contributions perpetrator programmes can make to victim safety as part of a coordinated community process. This is research which Respect themselves are currently carrying out.

In August 2010 Respect issued the following recommendations for perpetrator programmes:

1   Organisations operating without proactive (ex)partner contact or effective risk management should be considered unsafe.

2   Practitioners who are currently choosing to operate without these key elements need to suspend client work pending a review.

3   Agencies should avoid referring clients to services without these key elements and need to use their influence to try to persuade such services to suspend client work until these are in place.

4   Partners and ex-partners of perpetrators need to be informed about the dangers of their abusive partner participating in services that operate in unsafe ways. They need to be supported if their partner does not approach or participate in these services and offered information about their rights to protection and advocacy.

5   Referring agencies, funders, commissioners and others who have concerns about a particular agency offering perpetrator interventions need to ask that agency to provide information about their integrated support service and their risk management processes.
6   Referring agencies, funders and commissioners are recommended to contact Respect for further information about the appropriate standards or if they have concerns about perpetrator interventions that are not adhering to these safety issues.

They also suggest that programmes should be of at least 26 weeks' duration to help clients make sustained changes.

It is clear from this outline that Respect is a very important organisation providing guidance and research into perpetrator programmes and using international research to improve such programmes. They are robust guidelines and should be adhered to by all organisations providing perpetrator programmes.

Conclusion

It is clear from this discussion that perpetrator programmes are complex and need careful pre-programme assessment, that partners and ex-partners need to be engaged in the process, and that court mandated programmes provide better outcomes in terms of safety and controlling behaviour than voluntary programmes. The safety of women and children should be the core of these activities, as expressed by Respect. Many of the objectives outlined in the *Report of the Task Force on Violence Against Women* (1997) have not been achieved, and the lack of consultation with children who do not want to have contact with abusive fathers is very disconcerting. These are serious gaps in the provision of safety for women and children. Using the Respect guidelines is a clear way to ensure safety and protection for women and children. Engaging the court system to ensure that more abusive men are mandated to attend such programmes would also help outcomes and safety. Ensuring that the feminist model as outlined very clearly by the Duluth Model is also essential as it ensures that women are treated with respect and the Equality Wheel is kept in mind by programme facilitators. Controlling behaviour, as well as physical and emotional abuse, also needs to be kept in mind, as this is the core of domestic violence.

Bibliography

Abrahams, C. (1994) *The Hidden Victims: Children and Domestic Violence*. London: NCH Action for Children.

Ahmad, F., Riaz, S., Barata, P. and Stewart, D.E. (2004) 'Patriarchal Beliefs and Perceptions of Abuse among South Asian Immigrant Women', *Violence Against Women*, 10: 262–282.

AkiDwA (2008) *Understanding Gender-Based Violence: An African Perspective*. (Downloaded from: http://www.akidwa.ie/UGBV(November2008).pdf).

Alexander, H., Macdonald, E. and Paton, S. (2005) 'Raising the Issue of Domestic Abuse in Schools', *Children & Society*, 19: 187–198.

Allen, M. (2012a) 'Domestic Violence within the Irish Travelling Community: The Challenge for Social Work', *British Journal of Social Work*. 42 (5): 870–886.

Allen, M. (2012b) *Narrative Therapy for Women Experiencing Domestic Violence*. London: Jessica Kingsley Publishers.

Allen, M. and Forgey, M.A. (2007) 'Fuelling an Unnecessary Fire: Commentary on a National Study of Domestic Abuse in Ireland', *Administration*, 55 (3): 145–158.

Allen, M. and Forster, P. (2007) *Domestic Violence: Developing a Response*. Dublin: Exchange House.

Allen, M. and Perttu, S. (2010) *Social and Health Care Teachers Against Violence: Teachers' Handbook*. HEVI, University of Helsinki.

Allen, M. and Ni Raghallaigh, M. (in press) 'Domestic Violence in a Developing Context: The Perspectives of Women in Northern Ethiopia', *Affilia*.

Allen, M., Gallagher, B. and Jones, B. (2007) 'Domestic Violence and the Abuse of Pets: Researching the Link and its Implications in Ireland', *Practice* 18 (3): 167–181.

American Medical Association (AMA) (2005) *Report 7 of the Council on Scientific Affairs Diagnosis and Management of Family Violence*. (Downloaded from: http://www.ama-assn.org/ama/no-index/about-ama/15248.shtml).

Anderson, D.K. and Saunders, D.G. (2003) 'Leaving an Abusive Partner: An Empirical Review of Predictors, the Process of Leaving, and Psychological Well-Being', *Trauma, Violence and Abuse*, 4: 163–190.

Anderson, H. (1997) *Conversation, Language and Possibilities: A Postmodern Approach to Therapy*. New York: Basic Books.

Anderson, H. (2007) 'The Heart and Spirit of Collaborative Therapy: The Philosophical Stance – "A Way of Being" in Relationship and Conversation', in H. Anderson and D. Gerhart (eds), *Collaborative Therapy: Relationships and Conversations that Make a Difference*. New York: Routledge, pp.7–20.

Angus, L., Levitt, H. and Hardtke, K. (1999) 'The Narrative Processes Coding System: Research Applications and Implications for Psychotherapy Practice', *Journal of Clinical Psychology*, 55 (10): 1255–1270.

Archer, J. (2000) 'Sex Difference in Aggression between Heterosexual Partners: A Meta-analytical Review', *Psychology Bulletin*, 126: 651–680.

Asylum Aid (2002) *Romani Women from Central and Eastern Europe: A 'Fourth World' or Experience of Multiple Discrimination*. London: Refugee Women's Resource Project.

Bandura, A. (1973) *Aggression: A Social Learning Analysis*. Englewood Cliffs, NJ: Prentice Hall.

Bargai, N., Ben-Shakher, G., and Shalev, A. (2007) 'PostTraumatic Stress Disorder and depression in Battered Women: The Mediating Role of Learned Helplessness', *Journal of Family Violence*, 22: 267–275.

Barry, M.K., Bell, L., Devereux, P., Jordan, C., Lawlor, D., McCabe, C., McCann, S., Mooney, L., O'Rourke, A., O'Gorman, M., Valentyn, R. and Webster, K. (2010) *Practice Document on Domestic Violence. A Guide to Working with Children and Families*. HSE Dublin SouthWest Social Work Department.

Bateson, G. (1972) *Steps to an Ecology of Mind: Collected Essays in Anthropology, Psychiatry, Evolution and Epistemology*. New York: Chandler.

Bateson, G. (1979) *Mind and Nature: A Necessary Unity*. New York: Dutton.

Bauer, N.S., Herrenkohl, T.I., Lozano, P., Rivara, F.P., Hill, K.G. and Hawkins, J.D. (2006). 'Childhood Bullying Involvement and Exposure to Intimate Partner Violence'. *American Academy of Paediatrics*, 118: 235–242.

Beaulaurier, R.L., Seff, L.R., Newman, F.L. and Dunlop, B. (2005). 'Internal Barriers to Help Seeking for Middle-Aged and Older Women Who Experience Intimate Partner Violence', *Journal of Elder Abuse & Neglect*, 17 (3): 2005.

Bent-Goodley, T.B. (2005) 'Culture and Domestic Violence: Transforming Knowledge Development', *Journal of Interpersonal Violence*, 20 (2): 195–203.

Berger, P. and Luckmann, T. (1967) *The Social Construction of Reality*. Garden City, NY: Anchor Books.

Binney, V., Harkell, G. and Nixon, J. (1988) *Leaving Violent Men: A Study of Refuges and Housing for Abused Women*. Leeds: Women's Aid Federation England.

Birns, B., Cascardi, M. and Shannon-Lee, M. (1994) 'Sex-Role Socialization: Developmental Influences on Wife Abuse', *American Orthopsychiatric Association*, 64 (1): 50–59.

Black, D.A., Schumacher, J.A., Smith, S. and Heyman, R.E. (1999) *Partner, Child Abuse Risk Factors Literature Review*. National Network of Family Resiliency, National Network for Health (www.nnh.org/risk).

Bograd, M. (1999) 'Strengthening Domestic Violence Theories: Intersections of Race, Class, Sexual Orientation, and Gender', *Journal of Marital and Family Therapy*, 25 (3): 275–289.

Boonzaier, F. and de La Rey, C. (2003) '"He's a Man, and I'm a Woman". Cultural Constructions of Masculinity and Femininity in South African Women's Narratives of Violence', *Violence Against Women*, 9 (8): 1003–1029.

Bowker, L.H. (1983) *Beating Wife Beating*. Lexington, MA: Lexington Books.

Bowker, L.H., Arbitell, M. and McFerron, F.R. (1988) 'On the Relationship Between Wife Beating and Child Abuse', in K. Yllo and M. Bograd (eds), *Feminist Perspectives on Child Abuse*. Newbury Park, CA: SAGE, pp.158–175.

Bradley, F., Smith, M., Long, J. and O'Dowd, T. (2002) 'Reported Frequency of Domestic Violence: Cross Sectional Survey of Women Attending General Practice', *British Medical Journal*, 324: 1–6.

Bragg, H.L. (2003) *Child Protection in Families Experiencing Domestic Violence*. Washington, DC: US Department of Health and Human Services.

Breckenridge, J. and Ralfs, C. (2006) "'Point of Contact" Front Line Workers Responding to Children Living with Domestic Violence', in C. Humphreys and N. Stanley (eds), *Domestic Violence and Child Protection: Directions for Good Practice*. London: Jessica Kingsley Publishers, pp.110–123.

Brown, C. and Augusta-Scott, T. (2007) *Narrative Therapy: Making Meaning, Making Lives*. Thousand Oaks, CA: SAGE.

Brownridge, D.A., Chan, K.L., Hiebert-Murphy, D., Ristock, J., Tiwari, A., Leung, W. and Santos, S.C. (2008) 'The Elevated Risk for Non-Lethal Post-Separation Violence in Canada: A Comparison of Separated, Divorced, and Married Women', *Journal of Interpersonal Violence*, 24: 117–134.

Bruner, J. (1986) *Actual Minds, Possible Worlds*. Cambridge, MA: Harvard University Press.

Bruner, J. (1990) *Acts of Meaning*. Cambridge, MA: Harvard University Press.

Buckley, H., Skehill, C. and O'Sullivan, E. (1997) *Child Protection Practices in Ireland: A Case Study*. Dublin: Oak Tree Press.

Buckley, H., Horwath, J. and Whelan, S. (2006) *Framework for the Assessment of Vulnerable Children and their Families*. Dublin: Children's Research Centre, Trinity College and Sheffield: University of Sheffield.

Buckley, H., Whelan, S. and Holt, S. (2006) *Listen to Me! Children's Experiences of Domestic Violence*. Trinity College Dublin: Children's Research Centre.

Bui, H.N. (2003) 'Help-Seeking Behavior among Abused Immigrant Women: A Case of Vietnamese American Women', *Violence Against Women*, 9 (2): 207–239.

Bureau of Justice Statistics (2007) *Intimate Partner Violence in the U.S.* Washington, DC: Bureau of Justice Statistics.

Burke, J.G., Gielen, A.C., McDonnell, K., O'Campo, P. and Maman, S. (2001) 'The Process of Ending Abuse in Intimate Relationships', *Violence Against Women*, 7 (10): 1144–1163.

Burman, E., Smailes, S.L. and Chantler, K. (2004) 'Culture as a Barrier to Service Provision and Delivery: Domestic Violence Services for Minoritized Women', *Critical Social Policy*, 24 (3): 332–357.

Burton, S., Regan, L. and Kelly, L. (1998) *Supporting Women and Challenging Men: Lessons from the Domestic Violence Intervention Agency*. Bristol: Policy Press.

Burton, R., Baldwin, S., Flynn, D. and Whitelaw, S. (2000) 'The Stages of Change Model in Health Promotion Science and Ideology', *Critical Public Health*, 10: 55–70.

CAADA (2010) *Family Intervention Projects (FIPs) – Domestic Abuse Toolkit*. (Downloaded from: http://www.caada.org.uk/marac/TOOLKIT%20FIPs%20updated%20July%202010.pdf).

Campbell, D.W., Masaki, B. and Torres, A. (1997) '"Water on Rock": Changing Domestic Violence Perceptions in the African American, Asian American, and Latino Communities', in E. Klein, J. Campbell, E. Soler and M. Ghez (eds), *Ending Domestic Violence: Changing Public Perceptions/Halting the Epidemic*. London: SAGE, pp.64–87.

Campbell, J.C. (2002) 'Health Consequences of Intimate Partner Violence', *Lancet*, 359 (9314): 1331–1336.

Campbell, J.C., Oliver, C. and Bullock, L. (1993) 'Why Battering During Pregnancy?' *AWHONN's Clinical Issues in Perinatal Women's Health Nursing*, 4: 343–349.

Campbell, J.C., Garcia-Moreno, C. and Sharps, P. (2004) 'Abuse During Pregnancy in Industrialized and Developing Countries', *Violence Against Women*, 10 (7): 770–789.

Campbell, J.C., Rose, L., Kub, J. and Nedd, D. (1998) 'Voices of Strength and Resistance: A Contextual and Longitudinal Analysis of Women's Responses to Battering', *Journal of Interpersonal Violence*, 13 (6): 743–762.

Campbell, J.C., Webster, D., Koziol-McLain, J., Block, C., Campbell, D. and Curry, M. (2003) 'Risk Factors for Femicide in Abusive Relationships: Results from a Multi-site Case Control Study', *American Journal of Public Health*, 93: 1089–1097.

Carbonne-Lopez, K., Kruttschnitt, C. and Macmillan, R. (2006) 'Patterns of Intimate Partner Violence and Their Associations with Physical Health, Psychological Distress and Substance Use', *Public Health Reports*, 121 (4): 382–392.

Carlson, B.E., McNutt, L., Choi, D.Y. and Rose, I.M. (2002). 'Intimate Partner Abuse and Mental Health', *Violence Against Women*, 8: 720–745.

Cascardi, M., O'Leary, K.D. and Schlee, K.A. (1999) 'Co-occurrence and Correlates of Posttraumatic Stress Disorder and Major Depression in Physically Abused Women', *Journal of Family Violence*, 14: 227–247.

Casey, M. (1987) *Domestic Violence Against Women*. Dublin: Women's Aid.

Cawson, P. (2002) *Child Maltreatment in the Family*. London: NSPCC.

Cazenave, N.A. and Straus, M.A. (1979) 'Race, Class, Network Embeddedness, and Family Violence: A Search for Potent Support Systems', *Journal of Comparative Family Studies*, 10: 280–299.

Cemlyn, S. (2008) 'Human Rights and Gypsies and Travellers: An Exploration of the Application of Human Rights Perspective to Social Work with a Minority Community in Britain', *British Journal of Social Work*, 38 (1): 153–173.

Central Statistics Office (2002) Dublin: www.cso.ie.

Chang, J.C., Dado, D., Ashton, S., Hawker, L., Cluss, P.A., Buranosky, R. and Scholle, S.H. (2006) 'Understanding Behaviour Change for Women Experiencing Intimate Partner Violence: Mapping the Ups and Downs Using the Stages of Change', *Patient Education and Counseling*, 62: 330–339.

Children First: National Guidance for the Protection and Welfare of Children (2011) Dublin: Department of Children and Youth Affairs. (Downloaded from: http://www. dcya.gov.ie/viewdoc.asp?fn=%2Fdocuments%2FChild_Welfare_Protection%2Fchild first.htm).

Coates, L. and Wade, A. (2004) 'Telling it Like it Isn't: Obscuring Perpetrator Responsibility for Violent Crime', *Discourse and Society*, 15 (5): 499–526.

Cobbe, F.P. (1878) 'Wife Torture in England', *The Contemporary Review*, April: 55–87.

Cockram, J. (2003) *Silent Voices: Women with Disabilities and Family and Domestic Violence*. Nedlands, WA: People With Disabilities (WA) Inc. (Downloaded from: http:// www.wwda.org.au/silent7.htm).

Coker, A., Smith, P., Bethea, L., King, M. and McKeown, R. (2000) 'Physical Health Consequences of Physical and Psychological Intimate Partner Violence', *Archives of Family Medicine*, 9: 451–457.

Coker, A.L.L., Watkins, K.W., Smith, P.H. and Brandt, H.M. (2003) 'Social Support Reduces the Impact of Partner Violence on Health: Application of Structural Equation Models', *Preventive Medicine*, 37 (3): 259–267.

Coleman, K., Hird, C. and Povey, D. (2006) *Violent Crime Overview, Homicide and Gun Crime 2004/2005: Home Office Statistical Bulletin 02/06*, London: Home Office.

Coordination Action on Human Rights Violations (CAHRV): www.cahrv.uni-osnabrueck. de/.

COSC: The National Office for the Prevention of Domestic, Sexual and Gender Based Violence: www.cosc.ie.

Council of Europe (1950) *European Convention on Human Rights*. Rome: Council of Europe.

Council of Europe (2002) *Recommendation 1582 (2002): Domestic Violence Against Women*. (Downloaded from: http://assembly.coe.int/main.asp?Link=/documents/adopt-edtext/ta02/erec1582.htm).

Council of Europe (2008) *Stop Domestic Violence Against Women*. (Downloaded from: http://www.coe.int/t/pace/campaign/stopviolence/default_EN.asp).

Council of the European Union (2008) *EU Guidelines on Violence Against Women and Girls and Combating all Forms of Discrimination Against them*. (Downloaded from: http://www.consilium.europa.eu/uedocs/cmsUpload/16173cor.en08.pdf).

Council of the European Union (2010) *Council Conclusions on the Eradication of Violence Against Women in the European Union*. (Downloaded from: http://www.consilium.europa.eu/uedocs/cms_Data/docs/pressdata/en/lsa/113226.pdf).

1 Corinthians, 11: 3, 7–9. New Testament.

Cunningham, A. and Baker, L. (2004) *What About Me! Seeking to Understand a Child's View of Violence in the Family*. London, ON: Centre for Children & Families in the Justice System.

Currie, D.H. (1998) 'Violent Men or Violent Women? Whose Definition Counts?', in R. K. Bergen (ed), *Issues in Intimate Violence*. London: SAGE, pp.97–111.

Dasgupta, S.D. (2000) 'Charting the Course: An Overview of Domestic Violence in the South Asian Community in the United States', *Journal of Social Distress and the Homeless*, 9 (3): 173–185.

Dasgupta, S.D. (2005) 'Women's Realities: 'Defining Violence Against Women by Immigration, Race and Class', in N.J. Sokoloff, with C. Pratt (eds), *Domestic Violence at the Margins: Readings on Race, Class, Gender and Culture*. New Brunswick, NJ: Rutgers University Press, pp.56–70.

Debonnaire, T., Debonnaire, E. and Walton, K. (2004) *One Life Saved: An Evolution of Intervention Programmes in Ireland Working with Abusive Men and Their Partners and ex-Partners*. Dublin: Department of Justice, Equality and Law Reform.

Department of Health (1995) *Violence Against Women and Children*. (Downloaded from: http://webarchive.nationalarchives.gov.uk/+/www.dh.gov.uk/en/publichealth/violence againstwomenandchildren/index.htm).

Devaney, J. (2008) 'Chronic Child Abuse and Domestic Violence: Children and Families with Long-term and Complex Needs', *Child & Family Social Work*, 13 (4): 443–453.

Dobash, R.E. and Dobash, R.P. (1979) *Violence Against Wives: A Case Against the Patriarchy*. New York: The Free Press.

Dobash, R.E. and Dobash, R.P. (1985) 'The Contact between Battered Women and Social and Medical Agencies', in J. Pahl (ed), *Private Violence and Public Policy*. London: Routledge and Kegan Paul.

Dobash, R.E. and Dobash, R.P. (1992) *Women, Violence and Social Change*. London: Routledge.

Dobash, R.E. and Dobash, R.P. (eds) (1998) *Rethinking Violence Against Women*. Thousand Oaks, CA: SAGE.

Dobash, R.P. and Dobash, R.E. (2004) 'Women's Violence to Men in Intimate Relationships', *British Journal of Criminology*, 44: 324–349.

Dobash, R.E., Dobash, R.P., Cavanagh, K. and Lewis, R. (2000) *Changing Violent Men*. Thousand Oaks, CA: SAGE.

Domestic Violence: A Health Issue: Guidelines for Hospital Staff (2004) Dublin: St. Columcille's Hospital.

Donnelly, D.A., Cook, K.J., van Ausdale, D. and Foley, L. (2005) 'White Privilege, Color Blindness, and Services to Battered Women', *Violence Against Women*, 11 (1): 6–37.

Dowling, A. (1841) *Reports of Cases Argued and Determined in the Queen's Bench Practice Courts*. London: S. Sweet.

Dutton, M.A. (1996) 'The Battered Woman's Strategic Response to Violence: The Role of Context', in J.L. Edleson and Z.C. Eisikovits (eds), *Future Interventions with Battered Women and their Families*. London: SAGE, pp.105–124.

Edelson, J.L. and Tolman, R.M. (1992) *Intervention with Men who Matter: An Ecological Approach*. Newbury Park, CA: SAGE.

Edin, K., Dahlgren, L., Lalos, A. and Hogberg, U. (2010) '"Keeping Up a Front": Narratives About Intimate Partner Violence, Pregnancy, and Antenatal Care', *Violence Against Women*, 16: 189–206.

Ellsberg, M.C., Pena, R., Herrerra, A., Liljestrand, J. and Winkvist, A. (1999) 'Wife Abuse Among Women of Childbearing Age in Nicaragua', *American Journal of Public Health*, 89, 2: 241–244.

Ellsberg, M., Jansen, H., Heise, L., Watts, C. and Garcia-Moreno, C. (2008) 'Intimate Partner Violence and Women's Physical and Mental Healthealth in the WHO Multi-country Study on Women's Health and Domestic Violence: An Observational Study', *Lancet*, 371 (9619): 1165–1172.

Ellis, D. and DeKeseredy, W.S. (1997) 'Rethinking Estrangement, Interventions and Intimate Femicide', *Violence Against Women*, 3: 590–609.

Ephesians 5, 22–23. New Testament.

European Union (EU) (2007) Website of the European Union Commission. (Downloaded from: www.ec.europa.eu/employment-social/gender).

Fals-Stewart, W. (2003) 'The Occurrence of Partner Physical Aggression on Days of Alcohol Consumption: A Longitudinal Diary Study', *Journal of Consulting and Clinical Psychology*, 71: 41–52.

Fantuzzo, J.W. and Mohr, W.K. (1999) 'Prevalence and Effects of Child Exposure to Domestic Violence', *The Future of Children*, 9 (3): 21–32.

Farmer, E. and Owen, M. (1995) *Child Protection Practice: Private Risks and Public Remedies*. London: HMSO.

Farmer, E. and Moyers, S. (2005) *Children Placed with Family and Friends: Placement Patterns and Outcomes – a Report for the Department for Educational and Skills*. Bristol: Bristol University, School for Policy Studies.

Farry, N. (2012) Do Mandatory Groupwork Programmes for Perpetrators of Domestic Violence Increase the Safety of Women and Children? A Review of the North East Domestic Violence Intervention Programme. (UCD).

Ferguson, H. and O'Reilly, M. (2001) *Keeping Children Safe, Child Abuse, Child Protection and the Promotion of Welfare*. Dublin: A and A Farmer.

Fiebert, M. (1998) 'Annotated Bibliography: References Examining Assaults by Women on their Spouses/Partners', *Sexuality and Culture*, 1: 273–286.

Forgey, M.A. and Badger, L. (2006) 'Patterns of Intimate Partner Violence among Married Women in the Military: Type, Level, Directionality and Consequences', *Journal of Family Violence*, 21 (6): 369–380.

Foucault, M. (1980) *Power/Knowledge: Selected Interviews and Other Writings*, ed. C. Gordon. New York: Pantheon.

Freedom Programme: http://www.freedomprogramme.co.uk/index.php.

Gadd, D., Farrall, S., Lombard, N. and Dallimore, D. (2002) *Domestic Abuse against Men in Scotland*. Edinburgh: The Stationery Office.

Garcia-Moreno, C. (2002). 'Violence Against Women: Consolidating a Public Health Agenda', in G. Sen and P. Ostlin (eds), *Engendering International Health: the Challenge of Equity*. Cambridge, MA: The MIT Press, pp.111–42.

Garcia-Moreno, C., Jansen, H., Ellsberg, M., Heise, L. and Watts, C.H. (2005) *WHO Multi-country Study on Women's Health and Domestic Violence Against Women: Initial Results on Prevalence, Health Outcomes and Women's Responses*. Geneva: World Health Organization.

Garcia-Moreno, C., Jansen, H., Ellsberg, M., Heise, L. and Watts, C.H. (2006) 'Prevalence of Intimate Partner Violence: Findings from the WHO Multi-Country Study on Women's Health and Domestic Violence', *The Lancet*, 368 (9543): 1260–1269.

Gelles, R.J. (1974) *The Violent Home: A Study of Physical Aggression Between Husbands and Wives*. Beverly Hills, CA: SAGE.

Gelles, R.J. (1993) 'Through a Sociological Lens: Social Structure and Family Violence' in R.J. Gelles and D.R. Loseke (eds), *Current Controversies on Family Violence*. London: SAGE, pp.31–46.

Gelles, R.J. and Straus, M.A. (1988) *Intimate Violence*. New York: Simon and Schuster.

Gergen, K. (1991) *The Saturated Self: Dilemma of Identity in Contemporary Life*. New York: Basic Books.

Gibbons, J., Conroy, S. and Bell, S. (1995) *Operating the Child Protection System: A Study of Child Protection Practices in English Local Authorities*. London: HMSO.

Goddard, C. and Hiller, P. (1993) 'Child Sexual Abuse: Assault in a Violent Context', *Australian Journal of Social Issues*, 28 (1): 20–33.

Goffman, E. (1961) *Asylums: Essays in the Social Situation of Mental Patients and Other Inmates*. New York: Doubleday.

Goffman, E. (1974) *Frame Analysis: An Essay on the Organization of Experience*. London: Harper and Row.

Goldberg, C. (1999) 'Spouse Abuse Crackdown, Surprisingly, Nets Many Women', *The New York Times*, 23 November, A16.

Gondolf, E.W. (2002) *Batter Intervention Systems: Issues, Outcomes and Recommendations*. Thousand Oaks, CA: SAGE.

Gondolf, E.W. (2012) *The Future of Batterer Programes: Reassessing Evidence-Based Practice*. Boston: Northeastern University Press.

Gondolf, E.W. and Fisher, E. (1988) *Battered Women as Survivors: An Alternative to Treating Learned Helplessness*. New York: Lexington Books.

Goodman, L.A., Bennett, L. and Dutton, M.A. (1999) 'Obstacles to Domestic Violence Victims' Cooperation with the Criminal Prosecution of their Abusers: The Role of Social Support', *Violence and Victims*, 14: 427–444.

Goodman, L.A., Dutton, M.A., Weinfurt, K. and Cook, S. (2003) 'The Intimate Partner Violence Strategies Index', *Violence Against Women*, 9 (2): 163–186.

Goodman, L.A., Dutton, M.A., Vankos, N. and Weinfurt, K. (2005) 'Women's Resources and Use of Strategies as Risk and Protective Factors for Reabuse over Time', *Violence Against Women*, 11 (3): 311–336.

Gracie Productions: http://gracieproductions.com.au/Default.htm.

Graham, K., Bernards, S., Wilsnack, S.C. and Gmel, G. (2011) 'Alcohol May Not Cause Partner Violence But It Seems to Make It Worse: A Cross National Comparison of the Relationship Between Alcohol and Severity of Partner Violence', *Journal of Interpersonal Violence*, 26 (8): 1503–1523.

Graham-Kevan, N. and Archer, J. (2003) 'Intimate Terrorism and Common Couple Violence: A Test of Johnson's Predictions in Four British Samples', *Journal of Interpersonal Violence*, 18 (11): 1247–1270.

Graham-Kevan, N. and Archer, J. (2011) 'Violence during Pregnancy: Investigating Infanticidal Motives', *Journal of Family Violence*, 26: 453–458.

Grant, A. (1999) 'Resistance to the Link at a Domestic Violence Shelter', in F.R. Ascione and P. Arkow (eds), *Child Abuse, Domestic Violence and Animal Abuse*. W. Lafayette, IN: Purdue University Press.

Hague, G., Thiara, R. and Mullender, A. (2011) 'Disabled Women, Domestic Violence and Social Care: The Risk of Isolation, Vulnerability and Neglect', *British Journal of Social Work*, 41 (1): 148–165.

Haj-Yahia, M. (1998) 'A Patriarchal Perspective of Beliefs about Wife-beating among Palestinian Men from the West Bank and Gaza Strip', *Journal of Family Issues*, 19: 595–621.

Haj-Yahia, M. (2003) 'Beliefs about Wife Beating among Arab Men from Israel: The Influence of their Patriarchal Ideology', *Journal of Family Violence*, 18 (4): 193–206.

Hamberger, L.K. (2005) 'Men's and Women's Use of Intimate Partner Violence in Clinical Samples: Toward a Gender Sensitive Analysis', *Violence Against Women*, 20 (1): 131–152.

Hamby, S.L. (2005) 'The Importance of Community in a Feminist Analysis of Domestic Violence among Native Americans', in N.J. Sokoloff with C. Pratt (eds), *Domestic Violence at the Margins: Readings on Race, Class, Gender and Culture*. New Brunswick, NJ: Rutgers University Press, pp. 174–193.

Hammons, A. (2004) '"Family Violence": The Language of Legitimacy', *Affilia*, 19 (3): 273–288.

Harne, L. (2011) *Violent Fathering and the Risks to Children. The Need for Change*. Bristol: Policy Press.

Healthy Lives, Brighter Futures – the Strategy for Children and Young People's Health (2009) London: DOH/DCSF.

Hearn, J. (1998) *The Violences of Men: How Men Talk About and How Agencies Respond to Men's Violence to Women*. London: SAGE.

Hearn, J. (1994) 'The Organization(s) of Violence, Men, Gender Relations, Organizations and Violences', *Human Relations*, June, 47: 731–754.

Hegarty, K. and O'Doherty, L. (2011) 'Intimate Partner Violence: Identification and response in general practice', *Australian Family Physician*, 40 (11): 852–856.

Heise, L. (1998) 'Violence Against Women: An Integrated, Ecological Framework', *Violence Against Women*, 4 (3): 262–290.

Heise, L. and Garcia-Moreno, C. (2002) 'Violence by Intimate Partners', in E. Krug, L. Dahlberg, J.A. Mercy, A.B. Zwi and R. Lozano (eds), *World Report on Violence and Health*. Geneva: World Health Organization.

Heise, L., Ellsberg, M. and Gottemoeller, M. (1999) *Ending Violence Against Women*. Population Reports, Series L(11). Baltimore, MD: Johns Hopkins University School of Public Health, Population Information Programme.

Hester, M. and Radford, L. (1996) *Domestic Violence and Child Contact Arrangements in England and Denmark*. Bristol: Policy Press.

Hester, M. and Westmarland, N. (2005) *Tackling Domestic Violence: Effective Interventions and Approaches*. Home Office Research Study 290. London: Home Office.

Hester, M., Pearson, C., Harwin N., with Abrahams, H. (2007) *Making an Impact: Children and Domestic Violence*. London: Jessica Kingsley Publishers.

Heyman, R.E. and Smith Slep, A.M. (2002) 'Do Child Abuse and Interparental Violence Lead to Adulthood Family Violence?', *Journal of Marriage and the Family*, 64: 864–870.

Hicks, M.H. (2006) 'The Prevalence and Characteristics of Intimate Partner Violence in a Community Study of Chinese American Women', *Journal of Interpersonal Violence*, 21 (10): 1249–1269.

Hogan, F. and O'Reilly, M. (2007) *Listening to Children: Children's Stories of Domestic Violence Ireland*. The National Children's Strategy Research Series. Dublin: Office of the Minister for Children.

Holt, S. (2003) 'Child Protection Social Work and Men's Abuse of Women: An Irish Study', *Child & Family Social Work*, 18 (1): 53–65.

Holt, S., Buckley, H. and Whelan, S. (2008) 'The Impact of Exposure to Domestic Violence on Children and Young People: A Review of the Literature', *Child Abuse and Neglect*, 32: 797–819.

Home Office (2004) *Developing Domestic Violence Strategies: A Guide for Partnerships*. London: Home Office Violent Crimes Unit.

Hooks, B. (1990) *Yearning: Race, Gender, and Cultural Politics*. Boston, MA: South End Press.

Hotaling, G.T. and Sugarman, D.B. (1986) 'An Analysis of Risk Markers in Husband to Wife Violence: The Current State of Knowledge', *Violence and Victims*, 1: 101–124.

Hotaling, G.T. and Sugarman, D.B. (1990) 'A Risk Marker Analysis of Assaulted Wives', *Journal of Family Violence*, 5 (1): 1–13.

HSE Mid-West Area Adult Mental Health Domestic Violence Assessment Tool (2005). (Downloaded from: http://www.midwestvaw.ie/resources/recognise-respond-refer/respond/).

Humphreys, C. (2000) *Social Work, Domestic Violence and Child Protection*. Bristol: Policy Press.

Humphreys, C. and Thiara, R. (2002) *Routes to Safety: Protection Issues facing Abused Women and Children and the Role of Outreach Services*. Bristol: Women's Aid Publications.

Humphreys, C. and Stanley, S. (eds) (2006) *Domestic Violence and Child Protection: Directions for Good Practice*. London: Jessica Kingsley Publishers.

Humphreys, C. and Absler, D. (2011) 'History Repeating: Child Protection Responses to Domestic Violence', *Child and Family Social Work*, 16 (4): 464–473.

Humphreys J., Cooper, B.A. and Miaskowski, C. (2011) 'Occurrence, Characteristics, and Impact of Chronic Pain in Formerly Abused Women', *Violence Against Women*, 17 (10): 1327–1343.

Huth-Bocks, A.C., Levendosky, A.A. and Semel, M.A. (2001) 'The Direct and Indirect Effects of Domestic Violence on Young Children's Intellectual Functioning', *Journal of Family Violence*, 16 (3): 269–290.

Hyden, M. (1994) *Woman Battering as Marital Act: The Construction of a Violent Marriage*. Oslo: Scandinavian University Press.

Hyden, M. (1999) 'The World of the Fearful: Battered Women's Narratives of Leaving Abusive Husbands', *Feminism and Psychology*, 9 (4): 449–469.

Hyden, M. (2005) '"I Must have Been an Idiot to Let it Go On": Agency and Positioning in Battered Women's Narratives of Leaving', *Feminism and Psychology*, 15 (2): 169–188.

James, K., Seddon, B. and Brown, J. (2002) *Using It or Losing It: Men's Constructions of their Violence towards Female Partners*. Sydney: Australian Domestic Violence and Family Violence Clearinghouse Research Paper.

Jansson, K., Coleman, K., Reed, E. and Kaiza, P. (2007) *London Home Office Statistical Bulletin 02/07*. London: Home Office.

Jasinski, J.L. (2001) 'Theoretical Explanations for Violence Against Women', in C.M. Renzetti, J.L. Edleson and R.K. Bergen (eds), *Sourcebook on Violence Against Women*. London: SAGE.

Johnson, M.P. (1995) 'Patriarchal Terrorism and Common Couple Violence: Two Forms of Violence against Women', *Journal of Marriage and the Family*, 57: 283–294.

Johnson, M.P. (2006) 'Conflict and Control: Gender Symmetry and Asymmetry in Domestic Violence', *Violence Against Women*, 12: 1003–1018.

Johnson, M.P. (2008) *A Typology of Domestic Violence: Intimate Terrorism, Violent Resistance and Situational Couple Violence*. Boston, MA: Northeastern University Press.

Johnson, M.P. and Ferraro, K.J. (2000) 'Research on Domestic Violence in the 1990s: Making Distinctions', *Journal of Marriage and the Family*, 62: 948–963.

Johnson, M.P. and Leone, J.M. (2005) 'The Differential Effects of Intimate Terrorism and Situational Couple Violence: Findings from the National Violence Against Women Survey', *Journal of Family Issues*, 26: 322–349.

Jones, L.P., Gross, E., and Becker, I. (2002) 'The Characteristics of Domestic Violence Victims in a Child Protective Service Caseload', *Families in Society*, 83 (4): 405–415.

Jones, A.S., D'Agostino, R.B. Jr., Gondolf, E.W. and Heckert, A. (2004) 'Assessing the Effect of Batterer Program Completion on Reassault Using Propensity Scores', *Journal of Interpersonal Violence*, 19(9): 1002–1020.

Kantor, G.K. and Straus, M.A. (1990) 'The "Drunken Bum" Theory of Wife Beating', in M.A. Straus and R.J. Gelles (eds), *Physical Violence in American Families*. New Brunswick, NJ: Transaction, pp. 203–224.

Kasturirangan, A., Krishnan, S. and Riger, S. (2004) 'The Impact of Culture and Minority Status on Women's Experience of Domestic Violence', *Trauma, Violence, and Abuse*, 5 (4): 318–332.

Kaufman, J. and Ziegler, E. (1987) 'Do Abused Children Become Abusive Parents?', *American Journal of Orthopsychiatry*, 57: 186–192.

Kearns, N., Coen, L. and Canavan, J. (2008) *Domestic Violence in Ireland: An Overview of National Strategic Policy and Relevant Literature on Prevention and Intervention Initiatives in Service Provision*. (Downloaded from: www.Childandfamilyresearch.ie).

Kelleher and Associates with O'Connor, M. (1995) *Making the Links*. Dublin: Women's Aid.

Kelly, L. (1988) *Surviving Sexual Violence*. Minneapolis, MN: University of Minnesota Press.

Kelly, L. (1994) 'The Interconnectedness of Domestic Violence and Child Abuse: Challenges for Research, Policy and Practice', in A. Mullender and R. Morley (eds), *Children Living with Domestic Violence: Putting Men's Abuse of Women on the Child Care Agenda*. London: Whiting and Birch, pp. 43–56.

Kelly, L. (1995). *Crisis Intervention Responses to Domestic Violence*. Paper presented at St George's Conference, London.

Kelly, L. (1996). 'When Women Protection is the Best Kind of Child Protection: Children, Domestic Violence and Child Abuse', *Administration*, 44 (2): 118–135.

Kelly, L. (2005) *How Violence is Constitutive of Women's Inequality and the Implications for Equalities Work*. Paper submitted to the Equality and Diversity Forum Seminar, London. (Downloaded from: www.edf.org.uk/publications/LK_Equality).

Kelly, L., Bindel, J., Burton, S., Butterworth, D., Cook, K. and Regan, L. (1999) *Domestic Violence Matters: An Evaluation of a Development Project*, Research Study 193. London: Home Office.

Kewshaw, C., Budd, T., Kinshott, G., Mattison, J., Mayhew, P. and Myhill, A. (2000) *The 2000 British Crime Survey: England and Wales. Home Office Statistical Bulletin 18/100.* London: Home Office.

Khaw, L. and Hardesty, J.L. (2007). 'Theorizing the Process of Leaving: Turning Points and Trajectories in the Stages of Change', *Family Relations*, 56: 413–425.

Kildarestreet.com (2012) Dail debates, Tuesday, 13 March 2012: http://www.kildarestreet.com/debate/?id=2012-03-13.87.6.

Kimmel, M. (2002) 'Gender Symmetry in Domestic Violence', *Violence Against Women*, 8 (11): 1332–1363.

Kincaid, P.J. (1982) *The Omitted Reality: Husband-Wife Violence in Ontario and Policy Implications for Education*. Maple, ON: Learners Press.

Kirkwood, C. (1993) *Leaving Abusive Partners*. London: SAGE.

Kishor, S. and Johnson, K. (2004) *Profiling Domestic Violence: A Multi-country Study*. Calverton, MD: ORC MACRO.

Kitzmann, K.M., Gaylord, N.K., Holt, A.R. and Kenny, E.D. (2003) 'Child Witness to Domestic Violence: A Meta-analytic Review', *Journal of Consulting and Clinical Psychology*, 71 (2): 339–352.

Knox, J. (1558) *The First Blast of the Trumpet Against the Monstrous Regiment of Women*. Geneva: J. Crespin.

Kolbo, J.R., Blakely, E.H. and Engleman, D. (1996) 'Children who Witness Domestic Violence: A Review of Empirical Literature', *Journal of Interpersonal Violence*, 11 (2): 281–293.

Koran (1977), translated by J.M. Rodwell. London: Dent and Sons.

Krug, E.G., Dahlberg, L.L., Mercy, J.A., Zwi, A.B. and Lozano, R. (2002) *World Report on Violence and Health*. Geneva: World Health Organization.

Kurtz, D. (1993) 'Physical Assaults by Husbands: A Major Social Problem', in R.J. Gelles and D.R. Loseke (eds), *Current Controversies on Family Violence*. London: SAGE.

Leonard, K.E. (1999) 'Alcohol Use and Husband Marital Aggression Among Newlywed Couples', in X.B. Ariaga and S. Oskamp (eds), *Violence in Intimate Relationships*. Thousand Oaks, CA: SAGE.

Leonard, K.E. and Quigley, B.M. (1999) 'Drinking and Marital Aggression in Newlyweds: An Event-based Analysis of Drinking and the Occurrence of Husband Marital Aggression', *Journal of Studies on Alcoholism*, 60: 537–545.

Levendosky, A.A., Huth-Bocks, A.C. and Semel, M.A. (2002). 'Adolescent Peer Relationships and Mental Health Functioning in Families with Domestic Violence', *Journal of Clinical Child Psychology*, 31(2): 206–218.

Linton, J.L. (2002) 'A Prospective Study of the Effects of Sexual or Physical Abuse on Back Pain', *Pain*, 96 (3): 347–35.

Lipsky, S., Holt, V., Easterling, T. and Critchlow, C. (2004) 'Police-Reported Intimate Partner Violence During Pregnancy and the Risk of Antenatal Hospitalization', *Maternal and Child Health Journal*, 8 (2): 55–63.

Livingston, M. (2011) 'A Longitudinal Analysis of Alcohol Outlet Density and Domestic Violence', *Addiction*, 106: 919–925.

Lundy, M. and Grossman, S. F. (2005). 'The Mental Health and Service Needs of Young Children Exposed to Domestic Violence: Supportive Data', *Families in Society*, 86 (1): 17–29.

Luther, M. (1967) 'The Table Talk', translated and edited by T.G. Tappert, in *Luther's Works*, Vol. LIV, Philadelphia, PA: Fortress Press, p. 8.

McFarlane, J. and Parker, B. (1994) 'Preventing Abuse During Pregnancy: An Assessment and Intervention Protocol', *American Journal on Maternal Child Nursing*, 6 (19): 321–324.

McGahern, J. (2005) *Memoir*. London: Faber and Faber.

McGee, C. (2000) *Childhood Experiences of Domestic Violence*. London: Jessica Kingsley Publishers.

McKeown, K. and Kidd, P. (2003) *Men and Domestic Violence: What Research Tells Us*. Dublin: Department of Health and Children.

McLaughlin, J. (2003) *Feminist Social and Political Theory*. Basingstoke: Palgrave Macmillan.

McNeely, R.L. and Robinson-Simpson, G. (1987) 'The Truth About Domestic Violence: A Falsely Framed Issue', *Social Work*, 32, 485–490.

McWilliams, M. and McKiernan, J. (1993) *Bringing It Out in the Open: Domestic Violence in Northern Ireland*. Belfast: HMSO.

Macy, R., Ferron, J. and Crosby, C. (2009) 'Partner Violence and Survivors' Chronic Health Problems: Informing Social Work Practice', *Social Work*, 54 (1): 29–43.

Magowan, P. (2004) *The Impact of Disability on Women's Experiences of Domestic Abuse: An Empirical Study into Disabled Women's Experiences of, and Responses to Domestic Abuse*. ESRC/PhD Research, University of Nottingham.

Mann, J.R. and Takyi, B.K. (2009) 'Autonomy, Dependence or Culture: Examining the Impact of Resources and Socio-cultural Processes on Attitudes Towards Intimate Partner Violence in Ghana, Africa', *Journal of Family Violence*, 24: 323–335.

Marin, A.J. and Russo, N.F. (1999) 'Feminist Perspectives on Male Violence against Women', in M. Harway and J. O'Neil (eds), *What Causes Men's Violence Against Women?* London: SAGE, pp.18–35.

Martin, D. (1981) *Battered Wives*. San Francisco, CA: Volcano Press.

Martin, S.G. (2002) 'Children Exposed to Domestic Violence: Psychological Considerations for Health Care Practitioners', *Holistic Nursing Practice*, 16 (3): 7–15.

Melton, H.C. and Belknap, J. (2003) 'He Hits, She Hits: Assessing Gender Differences and Similarities in Officially Reported Intimate Partner Violence', *Violence Against Women*, 30 (3): 323–348.

Mental Health: A Report of the Surgeon General (1999). Department of Health and Human Services, U.S. Public Health Service (Downloaded from: http://profiles.nlm.nih.gov/ps/retrieve/ResourceMetadata/NNBBHS).

Mertin, P. and Mohr, P.B. (2002) 'Incidence and Correlates of Posttrauma Symptoms in Children From Backgrounds of Domestic Violence', *Violence and Victims*, 17 (5): 555–567.

Meuleners, L., Lee, A., Janssen, P. and Fraser, M. (2011) 'Maternal And Foetal Outcomes Among Pregnant Women Hospitalised due to Interpersonal Violence: A Population Based Study in Western Australia, 2002–2008', *BMC Pregnancy and Childbirth*, 11 (70): 1–7.

Miller, S. (2001) 'The Paradox of Women Arrested for Domestic Violence: Criminal Justice Professionals and Service Providers Respond', *Violence Against Women*, 7: 1339–1376.

Mirrlees-Black, C. (1999) *Domestic Violence: Findings from a new British Crime Survey Self Completion Questionnaire*. London: HMSO.

Mullender, A. (1996) *Rethinking Domestic Violence: The Social Work and Probation Response*. London: Routledge.

Mullender, A., Hague, G., Iman, U., Kelly, L., Malos, E. and Regan, L. (2002) *Children's Perspectives on Domestic Violence*. London: SAGE.

Myerhoff, B. (1982) 'Life History among the Elderly: Performance, Visibility, and Remembering', in J. Ruby (ed), *A Crack in the Mirror: Reflexive Perspective in Anthropology*. Philadelphia, PA: University of Pennsylvania Press, pp.99–120.

Nash, S.T. (2005) 'Through Black Eyes: African American Women's Construction of their Experiences with Intimate Male Partner Violence', *Violence Against Women*, 11 (11): 1420–1440.

National and International Statistics. (2012) Women's Aid. (Downloaded from: http://www.womensaid.ie/policy/natintstats.html).

National Children's Resource Centre (2003) (Downloaded from: http://www.cdc.gov/ViolencePrevention/intimatepartnerviolence/index.html).

Neimeyer, R.A. (1998) 'Social Constructionism in the Counselling Context', *Counselling Psychology Quarterly*, 11 (2): 135–150.

Neimeyer, R.A. (2000) *Lessons of Loss. A Guide to Coping*. Memphis, TN: University of Memphis.

Neimeyer, R.A. and Levitt, H. (2001) 'Coping and Coherence: A Narrative Perspective on Resilience', in C.R. Snyder (ed), *Coping with Stress: Effective People and Processes*. Oxford: Oxford University Press.

NIKK (Nordic Gender Institute): www.nikk.no/?module=Articles.

Nosek, M., Foley, C., Hughes, R. and Howland, C. (2010) 'Vulnerabilities for Abuse among Women with Disabilities', *Sexuality and Disability*, 19 (3): 177–190.

O'Faolain, J. and Martines, L. (1973) *Not in God's Image*. London: Temple Smith Ltd.

Ogrodnik, L. (ed) (2006) *Family Violence in Canada: A Statistical Profile*. Ottowa: Statistics Canada.

Osofsky, J.D. (1999) 'The Impact of Violence on Children', *The Future of Children*, 9 (3): 33–49.

Oxford Modern English Dictionary (1995) Oxford: Oxford University Press.

Pagelow, M.D. (1984) *Family Violence*. New York: Praeger.

Pahl, J. (ed) (1985) *Private Violence and Public Policy: The Needs of Battered Women and the Response of the Public Services*. London: Routledge and Kegan Paul.

Pavee Point and the Department of Justice, Equality and Law Reform (2005) *Challenging the Misconceptions of Violence against Minority Ethnic Women, including Travellers, in Ireland: An Information Brochure for Service*. (Downloaded from: http://www.nccri.ie/pdf/MinorityEthnicWomen05.pdf).

Payne, M. (2007) 'Narrative Therapy', in W. Dryden (ed), *Dryden's Handbook of Individual Therapy*. London: SAGE, pp. 401–423.

Peled, E., Eisikovits, A., Enosh, G. and Winstok, Z. (2000) 'Choice and Empowerment for Women Who Stay: Toward a Constructivist Model', *Social Work*, 45 (1): 9–25.

Pence, E. and Paymar, M. (1993) *Education Groups for Men Who Batter: The Duluth Model*. New York: Springer Publishing Company.

Perttu, S. and Kaselitz, V. (2006) *Addressing Intimate Partner Violence: Guidelines for Health Professionals in Maternity and Child Health Care*. Helsinki: University of Helsinki. (Downloaded from: http://www.hyvan.helsinki.fi/daphne/).

Pico-Alfonso, M.A. (2005) 'Psychological Intimate Partner Violence: the Major Predictor of Posttraumatic Stress Disorder in Abused Women', *Neuroscience and Biobehavioural Reviews* 29: 181–193.

Pittaway, E. (2004) *The Ultimate Betrayal: An Examination of the Experience of Domestic and Family Violence in Refugee Communities*. Occasional Paper 5. Sydney: Centre for Refugee Research: University of New South Wales.

Pleck, E., Pleck, J.H., Grossman, M. and Bart, P.B. (1977–78) 'The Battered Data Syndrome: A Comment on Steinmetz's Article', *Victimology: An International Journal*, 2: 680–683.

Povey, D. (2004) Crime in England and Wales 2002/2003: Supplementary Volume 1: Homicide and Gun Crime. Great Britain Home Office Research Development and Statistics Directorate Information and Publications Group.

Prochaska, J.O. and DiClemente, C.C. (1982) 'Transtheoretical Therapy: Toward a More Integrative Model of Change', *Psychotherapy: Theory, Research and Practice*, 19 (3): 276–288.

Prochaska, J.O., Velicer, W.F., Rossi, J.S., Goldstein, M.G., Marcus, B.H. and Rawoski, W. (1994) 'States of Change and Decisional Balance for 12 Problem Behaviours', *Health Psychology*. 13 (1): 39–46.

Radford, J. (2003) 'Professionalising Responses to Domestic Violence in the UK: Definitional Difficulties', *Community Safety Journal*, 2 (1): 32–39.

Rajagopalan, V., Price, P. and Donaghy, P. (2008) *An Evaluation of the East London DVIP*. (Downloaded from www.respect.uk.net).

Ramsay, J., Rivas, C. and Feder, G. (2005) *Interventions to Reduce Violence and Promote the Physical and Psychosocial Well-being of Women who Experience Partner Violence: A Systematic Review of Controlled Evaluations*. London: Department of Health.

Report of the Task Force on Violence Against Women (1997). Dublin: Office of the Tanaiste.

Respect: www.respect.uk.net.

Richardson, V. (2005) 'Children and Social Policy', in S. Quin, P. Kennedy, A. Mathews and G. Kiely (eds), *Contemporary Social Policy*. Dublin: University College Dublin Press, pp.170–199.

Roche, S.E. and Wood, G.G. (2005) 'A Narrative Principle for Feminist Social Work with Survivors of Male Violence', *Affilia*, 20: 465–475.

Rodriguez, M., Bauer, H., McLoughlin, E. and Grumbach, K. (1999) 'Screening and Intervention for Intimate Partner Abuse: Practices and Attitudes of Primary Care Physicians', *JAMA. The Journal of the American Medical Association*, 282: 468–474.

Roehl, J., O'Sullivan, C., Webster, D. and Campbell, J. (2005) *Intimate Partner Violence Risk Assessment Validation Study: The RAVE Study – Practitioner Summary and Recommendations: Validation of Tools for Assessing Risk from Violent Intimate Partners*. Research Report submitted to the U.S. Department of Justice. (Downloaded from: https://www.ncjrs.gov/pdffiles1/nij/grants/209732.pdf).

Rosen, K.H., Stith, S.M., Few, A.L., Daly, K.L. and Tritt, D.R. (2005) 'A Qualitative Investigation of Johnson's Typology', *Violence and Victims*, 20 (3): 319–336.

Rousseau, J.-J. (1762) *Emile ou de l'Education*, edited by F. and P. Richard, Paris, 1939.

Ruddle, H. and O'Connor, J. (1992) *Seeking a Refuge from Violence: The Adapt Experience: A Study of the Needs and Characteristics of the Users of the Adapt Refuge*. Limerick: Mid-Western Health Board.

Safe Ireland (2011) *Lifelines to Safety. A National Study of Support Needs and Outcomes for Women Accessing Domestic Violence Services in Ireland*. Athlone: Safe Ireland.

Saunders, B.E., Williams, L.M., Hanson, R.F., Smith, D.W. and Rheingold, A. (2002) *Functioning of Children with Complex Victimization Histories*. Paper presented at the annual meeting of the International Society for Traumatic Stress Studies, Baltimore, MD.

Saunders, D.G. (1988) 'Other "Truths" about Domestic Violence: A Reply to McNeely and Robinson-Simpson', *Social Work*, 33: 179–183.

Saunders, D.G. (2002) 'Are Physical Assaults by Wives and Girlfriends a Major Social Problem?', *Violence Against Women*, 8: 12.

Saunders, H. and Barron, J. (2003). *Failure to protect? Domestic Violence and the Experiences of Abused Women and Children in the Family Courts*. Bristol: WAFE.

Schechter, S. (1982) *Women and Male Violence: The Visions and Struggles of the Battered Women's Movement*. Boston, MA: South End Press.

Schröttle, M., Martinez, M., Condon, S., Jaspard, M., Piispa, M., Westerstrand, J., *et al.* (2006). *Comparative Reanalysis of Prevalence of Violence Against Women and Health Impact Data in Europe: Obstacles and Possible Solutions. Testing a Comparative Approach on Selected Studies*. (Downloaded from: http://www.cahrv.uni-osnabrueck. de/reddot/190.htm).

Schwartz, M.D (1987) 'Gender and Injury in Spousal Assault', *Sociological Focus*, 20: 61–75.

Schwartz, M.D. and DeKeseredy, W.S. (1993) 'The Return of the "Battered Husband Syndrome" through the Typification of Women as Violent', *Crime, Law and Social Change*, 20: 249–265.

Scott, J.C. (1985) *Weapons of the Weak: Everyday Forms of Peasant Resistance*. New Haven, CT: Yale University Press.

Sev'er, A. (1997) 'Recent or Imminent Separation and Intimate Violence Against Women', *Violence Against Women*, 3 (6): 566–589.

Shamai, M. and Buchbinder, E. (2010) 'Control of the Self: Partner-violent Men's Experience of Therapy', *Journal of Interpersonal Violence*, 25: 1338–1362.

Sobsey, D. and Doe, T. (1991) 'Patterns of Sexual Abuse and Assault', *Sexuality and Disability*, 9 (3): 243–259.

Sokoloff, N.J. and Dupont, I. (2005a) 'Domestic Violence at the Intersections of Race, Class, and Gender: Challenges and Contributions to Understanding Violence against Marginalized Women in Diverse Communities', *Violence Against Women*, 11 (1): 38–64.

Sokoloff, N.J. and Dupont, I. (2005b) 'Domestic Violence: Examining the Intersections of Race, Class, and Gender – An Introduction', in N.J. Sokoloff with C. Pratt (eds), *Domestic Violence at the Margins: Readings on Race, Class, Gender and Culture*. New Brunswick, NJ: Rutgers University Press, pp. 1–13.

Southall Black Sisters: http://www.southallblacksisters.org.uk/.

Speizer, I. S. (2010) 'Intimate Partner Violence Attitudes and Experience Among Women and Men in Uganda', *Journal of Interpersonal Violence*, 25: 1224–1241.

Stanko, E. (2000) 'The Day to Count: A Snapshot of the Impact of Domestic Violence in the UK', *Criminal Justice*, 1: 2.

Stanley, N. and Humphreys, C. (2006) 'Multi-Agency and Multi-Disciplinary Work: Barriers and Opportunities' in C. Humphreys and N. Stanley (eds) *Domestic Violence and Child Protection: Directions for Good Practice*. London: Jessica Kingsley Publishers.

Stanley, N., Miller, P., Richardson Foster, H. and Thompson, G. (2010) 'Children's Experiences of Domestic Violence: Developing an Integrated Response from Police and Child Protection Services', *Journal of Interpersonal Violence*, 26: 2372–2391.

Stanley, N., Miller, P., Richardson Foster, H. and Thompson G. (2011) 'A Stop–Start Response: Social Services' Interventions with Children and Families Notified following Domestic Violence Incidents', *British Journal of Social Work*. 41: 296–313.

Stark, E. (2007) *Coercive Control: How Men Entrap Women in Personal Life*. New York: Oxford University Press.

Stark, E. and Flitcraft, A. (1988) 'Women and Children at Risk: A Feminist Perspective on Child Abuse', *International Journal of Health Studies*, 18 (1): 97–119.

Stark, E. and Flitcraft, A. (1996) *Women at Risk. Domestic Violence and Women's Health*. London: SAGE.

Steinmetz, S.K. (1977) *The Cycle of Violence*. New York: Praeger.

Steinmetz, S.K. (1977/8) 'The Battered Husband Syndrome', *Victimology: An International Journal*, 2 (3–4): 499–509.

Stets, J.E. and Straus, M.A. (1990) 'The Marriage Licence as a Hitting Licence', in M.S. Straus and R.J. Gelles (eds), *Physical Violence in American Families*. London: Transaction Publishers, pp. 33–52.

Straus, M.A. (1977) 'Wife-Beating: How Common and Why?', *Victimology*, 2: 443–458.

Straus, M.A. (1979) 'Meansuring Intrafamily Conflict and Violence: The Conflict Tactics Scale', *Journal of Marriage and the Family*, 41: 75–88.

Straus, M.A. (1990) 'Social Stress and Marital Violence in a National Sample of American Families', in M.A. Straus and R.J. Gelles (eds), *Physical Violence in American Families*. London: Transaction Publishers, pp. 181–202.

Straus, M.A. and Gelles, R.J. (eds) (1990) *Physical Violence in American Families*. London: Transaction Publishers.

Straus, M.A., Gelles, R.J. and Steinmetz, S.K. (1980) *Behind Closed Doors: Violence in the American Family*. New York: DoubleDay.

Sugg, N., Thompson, R., Thompson, D., Maiuro, R. and Rivara, F. (1999) 'Domestic Violence and Primary Care: Attitudes, Practices, and Beliefs', *Archives of Family Medicine*, 8: 301–306.

Swan, S.C. and Snow, D.L (2002) 'A Typology of Women's Use of Violence in Intimate Relationships', *Violence Against Women*, 8: 286–319.

Swan, S.C. and Snow, D.L. (2006) 'The Development of Theory of Women's Use of Violence in Intimate Relationships', *Violence Against Women*, 12 (11): 1026–1045.

Swan, S.C., Gambone, L.J., Sullivan, T.P. and Snow, D. (2007) 'A Review of Research on Women's Use of Violence with Male Intimate Partners', *Violence and Victims*, 23 (3): 301–14.

Taft, A., Hegarty, K. and Flood, M. (2001) 'Are Men and Women Equally Violent to Intimate Partners?', *Australian and New Zealand Journal of Public Health*, 25: 498–500.

Testa, M., Quigley, B.M. and Leonard, K.E. (2003) 'Does Alcohol Make a Difference? Within-participants Comparison of Incidents of Partner Violence', *Journal of Interpersonal Violence*, 18: 735–743.

The Power to Change: How to Set Up and Run Support Groups for Victims and Survivors of Domestic Violence. (2008) Daphne project "Survivors Speak Up for their Dignity-Supporting Victims and Survivors of Domestic Violence, 2007–2009".

The Royal Australian College of General Practitioners (1998) *Abuse and Violence*. (Downloaded from: http://www.racgp.org.au/download/documents/Guidelines/2008abuseandviolence.pdf).

The Scottish Executive (2000) *The 2000 Scottish Crime Survey*. Edinburgh: The Stationery Office.

Thiary, R.K., Hague, G., Bashall, R., Ellis, B. and Mullender, A. (2012) *Disabled Women and Domestic Violence: Responding to the Experiences of Survivors*. London: Jessica Kingsley Publishers.

Tjaden, P. and Thoennes, N. (2000) 'Prevalence and Consequences of Male to Female and Female to Male Intimate Partner Violence as Measured by the National Violence Against Women Survey', *Violence Against Women*, 6: 142–161.

Todd, N. and Wade, A. (2003) 'Coming to Terms with Violence and Resistance: From a Language of Effects to a Language of Responses', in T. Strong and D. Pare (eds), *Furthering Talk: Advances in the Discursive Therapies*. New York: Kluwer Academic/ Plenum, pp. 145–161.

Tolman, R. and Wang, H. (2005) 'Domestic Violence and Women's Employment: Fixed Effects Models of Three Waves of Women's Employment Study Data', *American Journal of Community Psychology*, 36: 147–158.

United Nations (UN) (1995) *Beijing Declaration and Platform of Action, Domestic Violence Against Women*. Geneva: United Nations.

United Nations General Assembly (1993) *Declaration on the Elimination of Violence against Women*. General Assembly resolution 48/104 of 20 December 1993. (Downloaded from: http://www.wunrn.com/reference/pdf/Elimination_violence_women.PDF).

United Nations Population Fund (2000) *State of the World Population: Lives Together, Worlds Apart*. (Downloaded from: http://www.unfpa.org/webdav/site/global/shared/ documents/publications/2000/swp2000_eng.pdf).

UN Secretary-General (2006) *In-depth Study on all Forms of Violence Against Women*. (Downloaded from: http://www.un.org/womenwatch/daw/vaw/SGstudyvaw.htm).

Vieraitis, L.M. and Williams, M.R. (2002) 'Assessing the Impact of Gender Inequality on Female Homicide Victimization across U.S. Cities', *Violence Against Women*, 8 (1): 35–63.

Vogelman, L. and Eagle, G. (1991) 'Overcoming Endemic Violence Against Women', *Social Justice*. 18: 209–229.

Volpp, L. (2005) 'Feminism versus Multiculturalism', in N.J. Sokoloff with C. Pratt (eds), *Domestic Violence at the Margins: Readings on Race, Class, Gender and Culture*. New Brunswick, NJ: Rutgers University Press, pp. 39–49.

Wade, A. (1997) 'Small Acts of Living: Everyday Resistance to Violence and Other Forms of Oppression', *Journal of Contemporary Family Therapy*, 19 (1): 23–40.

Wade, A. (2000) *Resistance to Interpersonal Violence: Implications for the Practice of Therapy*. Unpublished doctoral dissertation. Victoria, BC: University of Victoria.

Wade, A. (2007) 'Despair, Resistance, Hope', in C. Flaskas, I. McCarthy and J. Sheehan (eds), *Hope and Despair in Narrative and Family Therapy: Adversity, Forgiveness and Reconciliation*. Hove: Brunner-Routledge.

Walby, S. and Allen, J. (2004) *Domestic Violence, Sexual Assault and Stalking: Findings from the British Crime Survey*. London: Home Office Research, Development and Statistics Directorate.

Walker, L.E.A. (1979) *The Battered Woman*. New York: Harper and Row.

Walker, L.E.A. (1984) *The Battered Woman Syndrome*. New York: Springer.

Walker, L.E.A. (1991) 'Post-traumatic Stress Disorder in Women: Diagnosis and Treatment of Battered Woman Syndrome', *Psychotherapy: Theory, Research, Practice, Training*, 28 (1): 21–29.

Walker, L.E.A. (1993) 'The Battered Woman Syndrome is a Psychological Consequence of Abuse', in R.J. Gelles and D.R. Loseke (eds), *Current Controversies in Family Violence*. Newbury Park, CA: SAGE, pp. 133–152.

Watson, D. and Parsons, S. (2005) *Domestic Abuse of Women and Men in Ireland*. Dublin: National Crime Council of Ireland.

Waugh, F. and Bonner, M. (2002) 'Domestic Violence and Child Protection: Issues in Safety Planning', *Child Abuse Review*, 11: 282–295.

Wenzel, S.L., Tucker, J.S., Hambarsoomian, K. and Elliott, M.N. (2006) 'Toward a More Comprehensive Understanding of Violence against Impoverished Women', *Journal of Interpersonal Violence*, 21 (6): 820–839.

White, M. (1989) *Selected Papers*. Adelaide: Dulwich Centre Publications.

White, M. (1995) *Re-Authoring Lives*. Adelaide: Dulwich Centre Publications.

White, M. (2000) *Reflections on Narrative Practice*. Adelaide: Dulwich Centre Publications.

White, M. (2007) *Maps of Narrative Practice*. New York: Norton and Company.

White, M. and Epston, D. (1990) *Narrative Ends to Therapeutic Means*. London: W.W. Norton & Company.

Wiist, W.H. and McFarlane, J. (1999) 'The Effectiveness of an Abuse Assessment Protocol in Public Health Prenatal Clinics', *American Journal of Public Health*, 89 (8): 1217–1221.

Wilcox, P. (2006) *Surviving Domestic Violence: Gender, Poverty and Agency*. Basingstoke: Palgrave Macmillan.

Wilson, M. and Daly, M. (1993) 'An Evolutionary Psychological Perspective on Male Sexual Proprietariness and Violence Against Women', *Violence and Victims*, 8: 271–294.

Wisner, C.L., Gilmer, T.P., Saltzman, L.E. and Zink, T.M. (1999) 'Intimate Partner Violence Against Women: Do Victims Cost Health Plans More?', *Journal of Family Practice*. 48: 439–443.

Women's Aid (2011) www.womensaid.ie.

Wood, G.G. and Middleman, R.R. (1992) 'Groups to Empower Battered Women', *Affilia*, 7(4): 82–95.

Wood, G.G. and Roche, S.E. (2001) 'An Emancipatory Principle for Social Work with Survivors of Male Violence', *Affilia*, 16: 66–79.

Wood, J.T. (2001) 'The Normalization of Violence in Heterosexual Romantic Relationships: Women's Narratives of Love and Violence', *Journal of Social and Personal Relationships*, 18: 239–261.

Wood, J.T. (2004) 'Monsters and Victims: Male Felons' Accounts of Intimate Partner Violence', *Journal of Social and Personal Relationships*, 21: 555–576.

Wood, R.C., McConnell, S., Moore, Q., Clarkwest, A. and Hsueh, J. (2010) *Strengthening Unmarried Parents' Relationships: The Early Impact of Building Strong Families*. Princeton, NJ: Mathematica Policy Research

World Health Organization (WHO) (2006). *Intimate Partner Violence and Alcohol*. (Downloaded from: http://www.who.int/violence_injury_prevention/violence/world_report/factsheets/ft_intimate.pdf).

World Health Organization (WHO) (2008). *A Global Response to Elder Abuse and Neglect: Building Primary Health Care Capacity to Deal with the Problem Worldwide: Main Report*. (Downloaded from: http://www.who.int/ageing/publications/ELDER_DocAugust08.pdf).

World Health Organization (WHO) (2010) *Expert Meeting on Health-Sector Responses to Violence Against Women*: (Downloaded from: http://whqlibdoc.who.int/publications/2010/9789241500630_eng.pdf).

World Health Organization (WHO) (2011) *Intimate Partner Violence During Pregnancy*. (Downloaded from: http://whqlibdoc.who.int/hq/2011/WHO_RHR_11.35_eng.pdf).

Yllo, K.A. (1984) 'The Status of Women, Marital Equality, and Violence Against Wives', *Journal of Family Issues*, 5 (3): 307–320.

Index